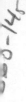

Review of Allied Health Education: 1

Review of Allied

Darrel J. Mase,
J. Warren Perry,
Associate Editors

Mary Dulmage,
Managing Editor

Health Education: 1

Joseph Hamburg,
General Editor

The University Press of Kentucky

This publication was supported in part by
NIH Grant 1 RO1 LM 01927-01 from the National
Library of Medicine

ISBN: 0-8131-1322-9

Library of Congress Catalog Card Number: 74-7876

A statewide cooperative scholarly publishing agency
serving Berea College, Centre College of Kentucky,
Eastern Kentucky University, Georgetown College,
Kentucky Historical Society, Kentucky State University,
Morehead State University, Murray State University,
Northern Kentucky State College, Transylvania University,
University of Kentucky, University of Louisville, and
Western Kentucky University.

Editorial and Sales Offices: Lexington, Kentucky 40506

CONTENTS

PREFACE

Several years ago a medical student on the campus of one of the editors set out to determine how much, or how little, his own faculty and fellow students actually knew about the burgeoning field of allied health. This was at a time when everyone in health education was beginning to talk about such things as health care teams and cooperative efforts at health care delivery.

So harrowing were his findings that they were never published. Among those who should have been best informed, the student discovered only a high level of ignorance.

By some stroke of luck, allied health faculty and students were omitted from the survey, thus sparing the editor a perhaps fatal blow.

We recount this sad tale, not to set a pessimistic or cynical tone but to point out that problems in communication harass all of us concerned with the education of health science students.

Allied health—perhaps because of its diversity, its youth, and its recent rapid growth and expansion—seems to be afflicted with more than its fair share of communication difficulties. Attempts are being made, however, to close some of the gaps, particularly at the academic level. The past decade has witnessed the birth of a new academic administrative unit—the college of allied health professions. Beginning in the early sixties, when fewer than fifteen such entities could be identified in the country, the number of allied health units has grown until today almost every major campus offers, under one title or another, a varied collection of such programs. This clustering of curricula has been of some help in improving understanding among faculty and students, but not as much as many of us had hoped.

As administrators responsible for directing these new educational structures at our respective universities, we believed that an understanding and appreciation of each team member's role and functions were essential—indeed critical—to the attainment of what we envisioned for the allied health professional. Instead, we daily confronted problems of poor communication between and among them.

Our vision perceived future health care as a team effort, of shared responsibilities among the practicing health professions, and that in this sharing the allied health professional would come to assume a much more important role than in the past. If this were to be, then it was imperative that members of these future teams begin to learn more about each other's competencies and capabilities. It was vital, as well, that they become aware of some of the broader and more general aspects of health care delivery.

Colleges or schools of allied health were providing the proper milieu for creating this new awareness, but there was still something missing: Allied health in general and allied health education in particular lacked a common literature. The scientific or academic activities of all these diverse disciplines were reported in the specialty journals of each, journals rarely read by professionals or educators outside the specialty. As a consequence, articles of common interest to a broad allied health readership seldom received proper exposure.

Those in education seemed to suffer more from this communication gap than the practitioners. In the kaleidoscopic arena of allied health education, curriculum innovation and experimentation were beginning to flourish. Many of these changes had relevance for other educators whose programs might profit from new approaches, yet there was little or no evident sharing of information.

It was from consideration of this void that the idea for this *Review* was born—a review that would provide a locus for articles of a broad and general nature which the entire spectrum of allied health educators and students might find of interest; a source book of current, discriminative information and opinion relative to the preparation of allied health professionals—written by persons of recognized and respected talent.

The University Press of Kentucky and the National Library

of Medicine were immediately receptive to the idea of producing such a publication, and it was with their encouragement and support that it becomes a reality with this first volume. Equally important was the enthusiasm of the scholars who were asked to contribute.

This first volume will, it is hoped, accomplish a three-fold objective: to give students, educators, and practitioners a new understanding of the work of other members of the health care team; to exchange ideas and information on innovative programs and practices in the field of allied health education; and to stimulate thought on what new directions we might take that will improve training programs and ultimately benefit the object of our common concern—the patient.

Obviously, one volume cannot cover in detail each allied health profession and all the issues related to health care and health care education. It is our intention to publish additional reviews on a regular basis, future volumes being devoted to other health disciplines as well as to general topics which we believe are important to all of us in allied health education.

Joseph Hamburg
Darrel J. Mase
J. Warren Perry

PREVENTIVE HEALTH CARE &
THE ALLIED HEALTH PROFESSIONS

Edmund D. Pellegrino

Disease prevention and health maintenance are inevitably included in any list of medical responsibilities. With equal inevitability, they are among the most neglected sectors of health care. Indeed, at no time and in no country have the available preventive measures been applied vigorously or to a whole population.

Today, more than ever before, we possess an extensive fund of reliable information about the prevention of some of our major ills. Were we to make effective use of this information on a wide scale, we could materially alter mortality, morbidity, and disability. Yet, we do not do so, and we are not likely to do so, without some major alteration in the organization of health care and the deployment of the specific functions of prevention to health professionals other than physicians.

ROOTS OF THE PRESENT DILEMMA

The reasons for the neglect of preventive medicine are relatively uncomplicated. They are rooted in the history of medicine and medical education, in the public expectations of physicians, and in the physician's traditional image of himself. The general public, understandably, has always been preoccupied with the availability of physicians for emergencies, acute illnesses, and the amelioration of chronic illness—in that order. There is, as yet, no public clamor for preventive medicine to equal the clamor for primary care or emergency medical services.

The physician has traditionally been trained to meet public expectations for curative medicine. The rewards and personal satisfactions derived therefrom are immediately tangible. His efforts in curative medicine are far more easily understood by society than the more frustrating efforts to change human behavior, which are the foundation of any satisfactory health maintenance program.

Dismaying as all of this may be, these factors are part of the reality of medical care, and there is every indication they will remain so. Unless many more physicians are available, accessible, and better distributed than they are now and unless some drastic alteration occurs in public and medical attitudes, we must look elsewhere than to the physician for the manpower requisite to mount a nationwide program of health maintenance and prevention. Even if we had a surplus of physicians, it is improbable that they would devote major efforts to prevention. Nor is it economically sound to rely on physicians trained for technical and diagnostic tasks, at great expense and over a long period, to provide preventive medicine, which requires different skills, attitudes, and knowledge.

The physician faced with the choice of curative or preventive medicine is forced to slight prevention before the genuine exigencies of acute medicine. Preventive measures are too important to be dependent upon the fortuitous attentions of a harried though "compleat" physician, however good his intentions and however genuine his interests. To force the physician to make this choice is not in the public interest, nor does it make best use of his training.

In actual practice, the more effective a preventive measure becomes, the less it requires the personal attention of the physician. Such obviously important preventive measures as vaccination, water and food sanitation, and chemoprophylaxis of malaria, for example, are most effectively applied to large populations by nonphysician health workers. The same can now apply to certain preventive aspects of personal health—like overnutrition, smoking, lack of exercise, abuse of drugs and alcohol—and to mental health. For prevention to be effective in these realms, the individual requires help in modifying his behavior by motivational reinforcement and a variety of educational and psychologic techniques for which many physicians do not have the time, the training, or the inclination.

Nothing in the approach we will discuss militates against the ideal physician who is dedicated to the practice of prevention along with cure. Every good physician, generalist or specialist, must combine both in some measure. The issue is not whether physicians should or should not practice preventive with curative medicine. Rather, it is whether this is a reliable basis for a nationwide program of preventive medicine. This essay argues that it is not, and proposes a viable alternative.

It seems reasonable from the above to conclude that a more realistic resolution of the deficit in preventive services is to assign the responsibility to a cadre of nonphysician health workers specifically trained for the tasks of prevention. Properly educated, properly situated in the health care team, and functioning as elements in a system of comprehensive service with the physician and other health professionals, such a cadre might permit us to apply what is already known for the benefit of larger segments of the population than is now the case.

Some Comments on Health, Maintenance, and Prevention

Before outlining who can best provide preventive services and under what conditions, we must arrive at some operational definitions of the three major terms in the discussion—health, health maintenance, and preventive services. This brief sojourn into the prickly territory of definitions is made without presumption and with the hope of providing some needed benchmarks for the rest of the essay.

The Concept of Health. Greek medicine, as exemplified in Plato and Hippocrates, explicitly aimed at more than the cure of disease. It held the cultivation of health to be an essential ingredient of the good life for the individual and for society. This was to be achieved by pursuit of a proper mode of living, and the physician was expected to assist the citizen in attaining this end. While medicine was not expected to confer immortality, it was expected to enable men to live a full life and to accept death in "due" time.

The precise definition of what constitutes health was as troublesome for the Greeks as it is for us. Yet, if it is to be an ingredient of a satisfying life, we need some clear definition of what it is we are seeking. The best we can hope for is an operational definition which, with all its deficiencies, will at least provide a benchmark for discussion.

The well-known definition of the World Health Organization is far too all-embracing. It equates health with complete well-being—physical, mental, and social. This would burden the health worker with the whole span of human concerns —from personal and community health to war, poverty, crime, and injustice. So global a task would discourage the most zealous and confirm the suspicions of the skeptics that the whole notion is vague and unattainable and, hence, safely ignored.

For our purposes, it is more useful to delimit the concept considerably. None of us is totally free of some physical, social, or emotional defect that in some measure impairs our satisfaction in living and our capacity to function optimally. We are all, in reality, located somewhere on a continuum extending from obvious disease and disability on the one hand, through absence of a discernible disease, to a state of optimum functioning at the other end. The continuum has physical, social, and emotional dimensions, and a person's health at any moment in time is the algebraic sum of these factors, which determine his location on the continuum. A person can only be healthy, then, in a relative and not an absolute sense—i.e., he occupies a position on the continuum that enables him to lead a satisfying life, to function in his chosen social role without significant impediment, and to enjoy some sense of well-being in all he does.

Health is, thus, a subjective as well as an objective state. It fluctuates constantly with the interaction of the cultural, social, physical, and emotional requirements of human existence. The continuum of which we speak is, therefore, not simply linear or even two-dimensional. It is, in fact, multi-dimensional and time dependent, as well. It is a positive concept and not simply the summation of a series of negative physical examinations, X-rays, or psychological tests. We can probably do little better in its definition than to fall back on the Greek concept of health as the fullest harmony between man's organism and his life situation.

Health Maintenance. The difficulties of defining health and determining the location of any individual on its multi-dimensional continuum are obvious. This complicates any definition of the idea of health maintenance. But here, too, we must attempt some operating definition.

The objective of health maintenance should be to sustain, preserve, and support a person's position on the health continuum. Maintenance, therefore, subsumes curative medicine and preventive medicine. Curative medicine has the task of aborting or reversing discernible abnormalities, thus bringing the patient back to the position he occupied on the continuum before becoming ill or, if possible, enabling him to better that position. Prevention aims at anticipatory intervention in the natural history of disease, forestalling the advance of established disease or avoiding its occurrence completely.

Health maintenance is, therefore, a comprehensive concept embracing curative and preventive elements. It must rest upon a close articulation of all elements within a health care system. To isolate or neglect any of these elements is to impair the notion of maintenance. Primary care, long-term care, secondary and tertiary care must be integrated with the modalities of prevention and positive promotion of health. Those who would establish separate systems of curative and preventive medicine would violate the unity of health maintenance and create a dichotomy, in the end injurious to personal and community health. This danger is particularly great in those romantic or embittered critics of medicine who call for prevention and even diagnosis and treatment to be separated from medicine entirely and turned over to "the people."

Clearly, if we accept the concept of the continuum, health and illness become dynamically interacting states. They can be disentangled functionally but must be kept in continuing contact with each other. Since persons cannot be classified as ill or healthy in any absolute sense, any organization of health services based on such distinctions opens itself to two alternatives—eventual duplication of the entire spectrum of services or rank neglect of one or the other element essential for an effective health maintenance system.

Preventive Services (Preventive Maintenance). Accepting the essentiality of an integrated system of health services, we can now deal with that portion of the spectrum of maintenance that is most properly preventive in nature. The essence of prevention, as noted above, consists in anticipatory intervention in the health care continuum, using knowledge of the natural history of health and disease to forestall or ameliorate disability or disease. Prevention encompasses three distinct subfunctions: 1) amelioration and containment of established chronic disease; 2) detection of unsuspected disease for which effective interventions are available; 3) prevention of the occurrence of new disease.

Each of these subfunctions deserves further definition, since each would be part of any effective program of health maintenance.

The first facet of preventive maintenance deals with containment of chronic diseases like heart failure, diabetes, arthritis, peptic ulcer, and respiratory, skin, and emotional disorders. The discomfort and disability that patients with such illnesses experience are controllable to variable degrees. The patients can be maintained in *relative* health by close medical supervision. Early detection of the signs of deterioration of function, a lapse in regimen, or a complication can reduce relapse rates for this large group of patients. The economic significance of effective disease containment is measured in prevention of hospitalization, as well as the reduction in days of disability and discomfort.

The second facet of preventive maintenance aims at the detection of unsuspected abnormalities by a variety of screening techniques. The advance of the discovered illness can be slowed by early treatment or specific education to help the patient modify his mode of life appropriately. Without entering here into the controversy about the cost/benefit relationships of mass screening programs, we can accept the fact that certain important disorders can be detected in this way. For these, early intervention can be important in keeping the patient healthy—i.e., early treatment of hypertension or bacilluria, overweight, dental and visual defects. When the current controversy over multiphasic screening is settled, it is reasonable to expect that certain screening measures will be found to be worthwhile. These, along with specific education and follow-up, will then become part of any sound health maintenance program in the future.

The third facet of preventive maintenance is primary prevention—preventing the first appearance of disease in an individual and even eliminating categories of disease entirely. This is the most rational and most effective modality of prevention, and it should be the ultimate aim of any responsible system of medicine. It includes a wide variety of measures: specific disease immunization, control of the quality of food, water, and air, control of chemical pollutants, noise abatement, and changes in life style, habits, and values detrimental to health—smoking, irrational use of food, drugs, alcohol, and automobiles, as well as patterns of destructive personal and social behavior.

This last category of preventive maintenance is the most difficult to apply on a wide scale and the least practiced. Yet, it holds the greatest promise for a reduction in some of the leading causes of mortality and morbidity. It is ultimately less expensive than curative or restorative medicine, and its potentiality for the positive promotion of the health of the entire population is still far from realization.

It is this last category, too, that least needs the physician's personal involvement and most calls for skills and educational experiences he may least possess. It is, in fact, the most promising sphere for the nonphysician cadre of health workers and one in which their contribution to the nation's health may be the greatest. Effective deployment of the tasks of prevention is a first step if we are to take advantage of the preventive elements of health care on a regional or national basis.

Deployment of the
Functions of Prevention

To meet the public mandate for health care that is accessible, available, comprehensive, humanely administered, and equitably distributed to all citizens requires optimal use of all existing and future health manpower. The dictum applies to all elements of health care and particularly to preventive services, in which newer patterns of organization are urgently needed. The tests of safety, utility, and efficiency should determine who best can perform a given function—not who may be doing it now or claiming perpetual hegemony over it.

We are beginning to see genuine attempts to distribute health care functions more efficiently among health professionals. In primary care, the physician's assistant, the family nurse practitioner, and the pediatric nurse practitioner have safely and competently assumed many of the physician's functions. Working cooperatively and under his supervision, they enable one physician to be available to more people, to cover a wider geographic area, and to gain time for activities that require his specific intervention. In tertiary care, the nurse on the coronary care unit interprets electrocardiograms and initiates treatment for arrhythmias, cardiac standstill, or acute heart failure. In chronic illness like hypertension and diabetes, the nurse or the physician's assistant assumes responsibility for patient management under predetermined medical protocols.

In preventive services, the tasks are now fragmented among a wide variety of professionals and nonprofessionals—physicians, nurses, dentists, pharmacists, health educators, physical educators, health cultists, and even charlatans. As a result, prevention—besides losing out in the competition with curative medicine—is also subject to duplication of some efforts, neglect of many others, and erroneous application in still others. Comprehensive, personalized preventive programs, based in individual needs and prescribed to suit those needs, are virtually nonexistent. Such services, however, constitute the essential basis of any effective national program of prevention.

Clearly, all practicing health professionals should be urged to add appropriate preventive measures to those particular segments of health care which they provide. Generalists, specialists, nurses, pharmacists, and allied health professionals can do much in the areas that pertain most closely to their points of contact with patients and the general public. Other health care personnel, specifically assigned the task of prevention, must work in cooperation with the major existing health professions in a mutually reinforcing relationship.

But the contributions of the physician and other health professionals now generally occur after a person has already become a patient, seeking help for some specific problem. Under these circumstances, prevention is apt to be limited to disease containment. While this is an essential element in an overall program of health maintenance, the real challenges lie in the spheres of early detection and primary prevention. These measures are most useful *before* the person becomes a patient, and their very purpose is to avoid that eventuality for as many people as possible. It is the provision of preventive services to those who consider themselves well that is most lacking and most in need of specific attention today.

Beginning in childhood and extending throughout life, there is need of available, accessible, feasible, and comprehensive programs to develop a more hygienic way of life based in the continuous practice of some simple but effective measures—a proper diet, low in saturated fats and adequate but not excessive in calories; regular physical exercise, abstinence from smoking, the use of all drugs parsimoniously for therapeutic purposes and not at all for nonmedical purposes, the limited use of alcohol, and other positive actions. To this basic regimen specific measures to guard against personal, industrial, and occupational hazards, inculcation of safe driving habits, better recreational habits, a monitored program of immunizations, and other safeguards should be added. At each stage in life there are specific needs for personalized preventive medicine, especially as they relate to emotional and social needs.

Our emphasis here is purposely on preventive personal health services. There are obviously many additional dimensions of prevention that are dependent upon the control of chemical and industrial pollutants of air, water, and earth; the hazards of travel, food processing, noise, etc. These also require our urgent attention if the personal measures are to have any real meaning. The design of a system to ensure a safe and healthful environment is beyond the scope of this essay, except insofar as modifications in personal habits and exposure can minimize the deleterious effects of the larger ecological milieu within which modern societies exist.

The precise content of a feasible program of personal preventive health services is yet to be defined. Whatever its content may be, two sets of preventive functions would seem to be desirable, each requiring different skills, capabilities, and educational preparation. Both sets of functions, however, can be performed by health professionals other than physicians and by being deployed among either existing or new health professionals. Without such deployment, preventive services cannot effectively reach the entire population.

The first of these sets of functions is predominantly of a technical nature. It consists of such tasks as the performance of periodic physical examinations and such specific preventive measures as obtaining Pap smears, breast and rectal examinations and proctoscopic examinations; taking routine histories, preparing health inventories and dietary histories; examination of sight and hearing, dental surveys, screening psychiatric and psychologic examinations, and a variety of other procedures involved in health assessment and disease detection. Included in this range of functions also would be the administration of standardized immunization programs for the entire population, according to a predetermined plan monitored by computer and supported by follow-up visit and education for those who fail to adhere to the prescribed regimen. Following protocols established by physicians and public health specialists, this cadre of technical preventive health workers would direct those with certain categories of findings to physicians for early treatment or to other preventive health workers for carrying out a personal preventive regimen based in the findings of the screening process.

In a properly integrated system of health maintenance, this

first category of function might be carried out by *preventive health assistants*. They would work in the same milieu as physicians, nurses, and others involved in curative and preventive care. They would work essentially with well people, acting as points of first contact for large segments of the population who would periodically be screened for specific categories of illness, both physical and emotional. They would also be responsible for maintaining a follow-up system, with periodic reminders and home visits to encourage the use of preventive services.

The second set of preventive health services would be of a more professional and less technical order, services associated with specific prescription and application of preventive health measures on a personalized basis, determined by the results of screening examinations performed by the preventive health assistants or by referral from physicians and nurses. Those performing this set of functions might be termed *primary health counselors*. They would also receive referrals from physicians, nurses, and other health professionals. Based on the recommendations of the physician, they would be responsible for the educational measures, health counseling, and behavioral modifications most appropriate for individual patients—dietary control, alcohol restriction, exercise—as the case may be. They would be expected to be skillful in educational methodology, small group dynamics, the techniques of motivational reinforcement and counseling.

These health counselors would assist people in following individualized preventive regimens, reinforced by group sessions and periodic follow-up examination. The workers in this category would be available for general counseling of all types, answering questions about current dietary fads, the utility of presumed preventive measures, and referring clients with incipient abnormalities or with technical and complex questions to physicians or other health workers.

These two categories of preventive health workers would require different educational preparation. The preventive health assistant would receive an education based in the more technical aspects of prevention and screening, most suitably at the associate degree level, with the usual admixture of general and technical studies. The primary health counselor would receive an education to the bachelor's level, emphasizing a more professional knowledge of the personal aspects of health education, counseling, small group dynamics, behavioral sciences, and the basics of mental health.

Preventive health services for children are of particular importance to the individual and to society. Both types of preventive health practitioners would be needed to work with pediatricians and pediatric nurse practitioners in office- and school-based preventive programs. They would concentrate their efforts on preventive health measures and maternal guidance during infancy and the earlier years of childhood. The special requirements of children with respect to immunizations, nutrition, growth and development, and emotional and social health within the family will require specific education for the preventive health technicians and counselors who will serve this age group.

One could envision a comprehensive health maintenance program based in the cooperative and integrated endeavors of physicians, nurses, and pharmacists working closely with these two specific categories of preventive health workers. Curative and preventive medicine could then be practiced side by side by individuals specifically trained for each, reinforcing each other, and providing continuity of curative and preventive regimens. Both types of preventive health workers could function in institutional settings, in physicians' groups, and in individual physician's offices. Both categories would be especially useful in health maintenance organizations (HMOs), industrial and community clinics, and other health agencies.

This close integration of preventive health workers with medical practitioners and other health professionals engaged in curative medicine would obviate the destructive dichotomy that has grown up between the practitioners of "health-oriented" and "disease-oriented" medicine. Such an articulation would make the continuum of health to which we referred earlier in this essay a reality, for the benefit of the patient and for the greater efficiency of the health professional.

The potential manpower sources for both categories of

preventive health workers we have described are plentiful and varied. First, those existing health professionals who now render preventive services part of the time could limit their efforts to this type of care. This would include public health nurses, health educators, and physician's assistants. Second, other health professionals, after additional training, could transfer to this type of work—e.g., pharmacists or social workers. Third, both categories can be educated from high school on, specifically for the tasks of prevention. Last, some of the surplus of college graduates in the social sciences, the humanities, and education could qualify for either of the two roles after a year or so of additional training. New job opportunities are urgently needed for the large number of such graduates (more than 500,000 in 1973) who now have difficulty finding suitable employment. Preventive health work would give them a satisfying outlet, use their educational experiences, and meet the desire of many of them to "work with people" and do something "meaningful."

The extent of supplementary education needed for those who move from other fields into preventive health work will vary with the content of their prior experiences and education. Clearly, once the decision to undertake a nationwide program of preventive health services is made, the necessary manpower cadre can be developed quickly and expeditiously.

CONVERGENCE OF FUNCTIONS
IN THE HEALTH PROFESSIONS

An immediate and justifiable objection to these proposals for improving preventive health services is that they will accentuate the duplication of effort and the fragmentation of health care, which now seriously plague the health field. Instead of multiplying health professionals, we should concentrate on condensing their functions in the interests of the efficiency, efficacy, cost, and comprehensiveness of the services they provide.

This problem is a particularly lively one in the field of preventive services, which are indeed fragmented, overlapping, and have little continuity. Figure 1 lists some of the

Figure 1

*Possible Patterns of Convergence of
Functions in Preventive Health Care*

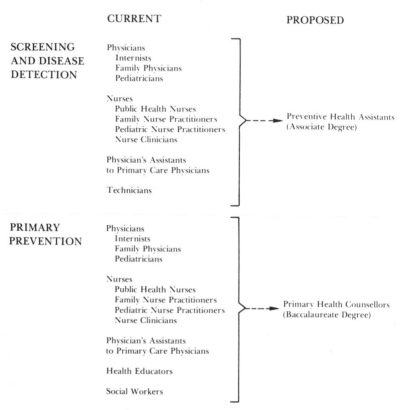

professions that now provide some modicum of prevention, with varying degrees of intensity and capability. No one of these professions has full responsibility in the health arena for preventive services. With few exceptions (public health nurse, health educator), most of the existing professions must divide their time between curative and preventive duties. Emphasis must, in consequence, be on the care of *patients* and not on the presumably well person who would like to avoid being a patient and to enhance his state of health by a more hygienic pattern of life. The resultant pattern of prevention is discontinuous, incomplete, and without adequate follow-up.

A reasonable solution to this dilemma is to effect some convergence of the fragmented functions into the two sets proposed here. Figure 1 suggests a way in which this convergence can be achieved. The primary responsibilities for preventive health services in the health care team would be redeployed to the two new categories, the one technical and the other professional. Those who now provide such services for part of their time would be freed to devote their full energies to curative medicine; those now providing these services who wish to enlarge their interests in preventive medicine would transfer to either of the new categories. No profession need lose its professional identity; rather, it would gain a significant new functional identity.

Of course, such redeployment raises many questions and anxieties crucial to the self-image and identity of the existing professions. While difficult, these questions can be resolved if the major focus is upon the needs of patients and society and if it is understood that some convergence of functions must eventually occur in all segments of the health care field. There is today an equally confusing duplication and fragmentation of services in the curative realm. All the health professions must sooner or later engage in a mutual, cooperative redefinition of functions based in the needs of those they serve, unimpeded by the jurisdictional prerogatives that now obstruct the efficient satisfaction of those needs.

This is one of the most pressing problems before us, the health professions as a group. Indeed, without its resolution, we cannot hope to provide rational answers about the types and numbers of manpower needed in the health professions now or in the future. Without these data, rational planning for service and education is impossible. As a result, those responsible for public policy are forced to make their own manpower estimates, which are apt to be less well-informed than if they were constructed out of the mutual efforts of health professionals. Unless health providers are able to transcend their parochial interests in the interest of the public good, they can expect manpower projections to be imposed by external forces.

Each profession must also limit its pretensions somewhat.

The ideal of each practitioner as a "compleat" or comprehensive professional for the "whole patient" bears more critical scrutiny than it receives. In the excruciatingly difficult task of reexamining its own role, each health profession must sincerely ask whether it can really practice genuine preventive care in addition to its other duties; or would it not be more honest to admit that only a limited portion of the spectrum of preventive services can be provided and that full justice can be accorded preventive care only by new team members who will assume primary responsibility for its practice.

The decisions to redeploy preventive functions and to effect the convergence of which we have spoken could be the beginning of a more searching reexamination of all the functions of patient care. This reexamination, if conducted rigorously and conscientiously, would undoubtedly lead to a regrouping of the whole spectrum of health professions into a smaller number, based in the fundamental categories of patients' needs and the levels of knowledge and skill required to satisfy those needs. The effort in the realm of preventive services could therefore serve two important purposes: first, it could provide, for the first time, a national program of preventive health services; second, it could illustrate how all other segments of the spectrum of patient care might be reexamined to meet the same needs for convergence and condensation.

The endless replication of new health professions to meet neglected areas of need or make up for the deficiencies of existing professions is socially and economically unacceptable. Some new ordering principles are required that will produce fewer categories of health professionals, based more firmly in the categories of patient needs. This is the only antidote to the uninhibited desires of old professions to retain all prerogatives, even if unexercised, or of new professions to fill neglected areas without reference to some coordinated plan in which manpower needs and patient care needs are made congruent with each other. We do not now have an accepted ordering principle. This is one of the exciting challenges the allied health professions and the older health professions can meet together in the next decade.

SUMMARY

The promotion of health and its maintenance have never enjoyed the same emphasis as the cure of illness, either professionally or socially. As we move, however haltingly, to the design of a national health policy, preventive health services must become an integral part of the spectrum of services available to all citizens. Otherwise, our nation would be denied the social, economic, and personal benefits that can accrue from the application of the knowledge we now have of disease prevention.

A comprehensive, personalized, and continuous set of preventive services can be provided by the deployment of the tasks of prevention to members of the health care team specifically trained for those tasks. Two categories are required, one technical and the other professional. The functions of prevention, now fragmented among a variety of professions, can converge in these two. Curative and preventive medicine can be better integrated within the health care team, each receiving primary attention from professionals dedicated and educated to meet the differing requirements of these two modalities of the total spectrum of health care.

Assignment of the tasks of prevention sharpens the larger issue of the optimal redeployment of all the functions of patient care among existing and new health professionals. The principles of convergence of functions and condensation of categories must eventually be applied to the whole range of medical and health care. The urgency of this responsibility and the challenges it provides can be met only with a cooperative effort among all health professionals. Such an effort is indispensable to a restoration of public confidence and to the evolution of any rational national plan for health care that meets the tests of equity, quality, and economic viability.

NOTES

This essay is a modification and extension of the author's 1971 James Fenton Distinguished Lecture, "Health Maintenance: An Idea in Search of an Organization," delivered at the State University of New York at Buffalo on October 20, 1971 and published in the *Proceedings of the Institute on Health Maintenance: Challenge for the Allied Health Professions* (Buffalo: State University of New York: Faculty of Health Sciences, 1972), 13-29.

For additional reading see E. D. Pellegrino, "Acute and Chronic Illness in the United States," *The Greater Medical Profession*. Report of a Symposium Sponsored Jointly by the Royal Society of Medicine and the Josiah Macy, Jr. Foundation. (New York: The Josiah Macy, Jr. Foundation, 1973), 57-72.

EDUCATION IN THE HEALTH & HELPING PROFESSIONS:

PHILOSOPHIC CONTEXT, MULTIDISCIPLINARY TEAM MODELS, & CULTURAL COMPONENTS

Marceline E. Jaques & J. Warren Perry

A continuum of health services available for human health needs, wherever and whenever they occur, stands as an ideal in the health professions. In fact, the ideas of caring for, treating, and preventing illness and disability, promoting and maintaining a healthy state of physical, mental, and social well-being are among the great hopes and goals that draw us together. Such states we want for ourselves and for people everywhere. Comprehensiveness and continuity of care have historically been inherent in the rehabilitation concept.

The reality in practice, however, is that we are far from achieving these lofty goals. We have, though, most of the capabilities and the skills available if we can decide on health as a priority, effectively organize resources, and educate and train manpower and womanpower to achieve it. The World Health Organization's definition of health is in the absolute terms of complete well-being in physical, mental, and social spheres of life. Pellegrino, however, takes issue with this concept of health as not existing in actuality.[1] He proposes an operational definition based on optimal functioning in a social role. Health in this context is more than absence of disease or disability, but is a positive changing state "measured in terms of satisfaction, productivity, and the enhancement of potentiality of the person."

Components of Health
Maintenance

To maintain health in this comprehensive sense involves the three major components of 1) treatment of illness and disability; 2) prevention of new diseases through early and regular detection; and 3) primary prevention through personal and environmental controls such as immunizations, proper diets, avoidance of smoking, alcohol, drugs, and accident prevention. One component is not sufficient unto itself. They are inter-related, and together, result in a system of health maintenance. Just as the goals are comprehensive, so must also be the patterns of service delivery. The traditional health and helping professions and professionals need to come together to find new ways of meeting consumer needs. Involved as equal partners—with multi-health professionals representing all areas and levels of education, knowledge, and experience—will be individual health consumers active in carrying out their own program of health maintenance.

This requires, likewise, a broad definition of "workers" to include not only the traditional medical and therapeutic disciplines, but also the helping professions such as rehabilitation counseling, social work, and psychology. A career ladder concept within these disciplines made up of support personnel (allied health and paraprofessionals), trained at two-year college and baccalaureate levels articulated to work with graduate level professionals, is essential to fulfill the objectives.[2]

Support personnel, often closer to consumer life style, are needed to perform tasks that the typical professional may find difficult. Communication and understanding brought about by the experience of sharing a problem or life style brings a reality and perspective not otherwise available. For example, perhaps the experience of coping with the problem of alcoholism may be understood in all its depth most fully by someone who has shared this type of problem.

Support persons are needed also to supply the quantity of health and helping persons needed in the total health and rehabilitation fields. We can neither supply the numbers nor afford the costs of training above the level of expertise needed to fulfill task demands. The development of more manpower to respond to the health needs of a country is crucial, but the magnitude or quantity of workers alone will never solve the problems faced. Rather, more effective utilization of the workers we have, coupled with inter-disciplinary systems of working together, have to become our primary goals in both education and practice.

The American health system has both priced itself out of the market and failed to deliver services needed by consumers. We hope other countries may profit from some of the errors we have made in this struggle to evolve a workable system.

The career ladder approach permits persons to enter with little training and education and progress up the ladder with more education and experience. This plan also helps handle the very complicated problem of the generalist versus the specialist in knowledge or skill. Ideally, everyone should be a generalist, perhaps, but to keep up with increasing knowledge makes this progressively more difficult.

Health information and service centers are needed in the community, close to the individual consumer's home and available when needed in a form useful and helpful for the problems faced. Hospitals, of course, will always be needed. But much of the service pressure, not of an acute nature, ordinarily put on hospitals can be relieved by other agencies such as community centers, nursing homes, half-way houses, and other forms of transitional housing. The goal is increasing independence for the consumer and appropriate utilization of personnel, facilities, and services.

Historically, care has been sought and provided only when illness or disability assumes crisis proportions, and while emergencies will always exist, a health maintenance concept assumes early intervention to be of primary importance. Such a shifting of emphasis to early detection and prevention of problems before they are of a crisis or emergency nature presupposes changes in attitude and behavior on the part of both the individual consumers and the professions.

Consumer and Self-Help

Working within the health maintenance concept, the consumer will not be passively "acted on" as a one-way recipient of service but rather considered to have inherent resources within, essential to the total effort. The use of the term *consumer* rather than *patient* or *client* assumes a partnership, and a joint team membership. Resources of the individual consumer need to be mobilized and used in directions of self-help. Care systems of the past have reinforced consumer dependency and frequently did not utilize or involve the individual and the family or the community as positive resources. The goal of all health and rehabilitation professionals should be to work themselves out of a job as soon as possible and permit individuals to actively collaborate in developing a system to sustain and maintain their physical and mental health. Along with the more traditional professional services, programs of health education, individual and group counseling are needed, as well as organized plans for self-help.

Two excellent examples of self-help organizations which have pioneered and amply demonstrated the efficacy of the self-help model are Alcoholics Anonymous[3] and Recovery, Incorporated.[4] These groups are now active worldwide and have helped thousands of individuals and families with problems of alcoholism and mental and nervous conditions. The group methods used literally permit persons who share experiences and problems to help each other to find help for themselves in the process.

Such self-help groups are growing in number with the concept spreading to include persons facing other problems or conditions such as addiction, mental retardation, colostomy, laryngotomy, cerebral palsy, and paraplegia, to name only a few. Families and friends are usually included or have groups of their own, such as Alanon for families and friends of alcoholics, and Alateens for children of alcoholics. The effectiveness of the process seems to involve both therapeutic and educational dimensions such as: 1) gaining facts and knowledge of the condition; 2) learning coping mechanism from those who are successfully living with the problem; 3)

gaining motivation and support from others who have shared
a similar life experience; 4) providing reinforcement through
the modeling effect of successful problem-solving, both for
new members and for long-term members; 5) self-evaluation
of progress from contact among members at various stages of
problem, knowledge, and levels of coping behavior; and 6)
identification with the group and development of a tangible
sense of belonging, both of an individual and social nature,
serving to minimize isolation and alienation.

THE HEALTH PROFESSIONAL

The education of health professionals designed to achieve
objectives of health maintenance needs careful reevaluation
of both past efforts and future goals. In the past, and in most
cases up to the present day, basic education has been aimed at
treatment and care through single modalities and the goals of
early detection and prevention have not been emphasized.
Therefore, students are primarily schooled in treatment
techniques in one area—their own. Too little understanding
of other disciplines exists, inter-professional communication
is at a minimum, and the consumer as an equal partner is at
best given lip service. Professionals are basically schooled in
the theory and techniques of their own fields, with little emphasis given to the development of interpersonal and interprofessional communication skills and experience.

The assumption seems to be made that these skills come
naturally and do not need emphasis during formal education.
It is our contention that this is not so, and that specific focus is
needed on the communication group process involved in
working together during the initial education and training
period. To carry out goals of health maintenance as defined
here requires collaboration of many disciplines—not only of
traditional health fields, primarily from the physical science
disciplines—but also from the helping professions, including
practitioners educated in the behavioral and social sciences.
This includes the basic disciplines of rehabilitation counseling, social work, psychology, and psychiatry oriented primarily to community practice.

The health professions are usually defined as including medicine, dentistry, nursing, pharmacy, and all allied health fields. Some allied health lists include as many as 200 fields, among them are the professions of dental hygiene; dietetics; inhalation, occupational, physical and respiratory therapy; medical records administration; medical technology; and radiologic technology. Health education and the disciplines of sociology and anthropology are needed to educate effectively such broad-based and multi-skilled workers.

We are faced with the dilemma of burgeoning knowledge and specialization in all professional areas. At the same time, professionals with a generic base are needed so that practice can be unified and whole. At present, professions are too often split one from the other, with the roots of the split deep in philosophy, knowledge base, and practice.

Mind-Body Dualism

The age-old dualism in Western thought of splitting the individual into two separate, yet interacting parts—body and mind—started with Descartes' philosophy in the seventeenth century and continues into modern psychology.[5] Eastern cultures and their philosophies, however, have not categorized mind, matter, soul, and body in the same way as have Western schools of thought. Though the cultures of Asia never gained the exacting physical knowledge of modern Western cultures, they grasped the holism of life in a way that is now occurring in the West. The organismic, (Goldstein, 1959),[6] to humanistic (Maslow, 1962;[7] Goble, 1970[8]), and Gestalt theories (Perls, Hefferline and Goodman, 1951;[9] Perls, 1969[10]) in the Western world have centered on the wholeness of the human organism and its life experience. These points of view bear likeness to Zen Buddhism in which the essence of *being* is explained in the individual's own totality of experience.

Most definitions and concepts of disability and illness have assumed, however, a dichotomy between the body and the mind. The body-mind problem is pervasive in the approach and development of the Western physical sciences and in most of the social and psychological areas of knowledge. The scientific method, though responsible for our vast knowledge pool, has also produced the practice of breaking problems into component parts for study and then studying each component separately. Little attempt to relate to other components has resulted in fragmented knowledge of the whole human being as an entity or a system. But each human part is related to other parts, and concepts that do not include this relatedness or wholeness of the human organism are incomplete. For when a person hurts or is sick or disabled, all aspects of his being, the whole of his mind and body, are affected and react.

This basic mind-body split has not only produced separateness in areas of knowledge, but has resulted in a proliferation of professional and technical practitioners. Emerging as they have from the separate knowledge bases, too often without a common language or a method of collaboration, the focus in practice on human wholeness is sporadic at best. The philosophic assumptions and concepts of rehabilitation have always focused on the holistic nature of man. An operational application of this holism has been the development and use of the team concept in rehabilitation practice (Jaques, 1970).[11]

But, to the dismay of most professionals, the team concept too rarely functions in a satisfactory way as a problem-solving technique. For in addition to the problems produced by separateness of knowledge base and practice methods, a hierarchical social status system among the professions influences the behavior of team members, both in response to each other generally and in group or team interaction. The professional hierarchy assigns status by type of profession, amount and kind of education and experience. Within the Western societies, particularly the United States, the physician is assigned the highest status, followed on a descending scale, by doctoral level education in other fields; masters, baccalaureate, and associate degrees; certificates; and lesser amounts of schooling. Experience counts for less status than education, technical skills for less than theoretical knowledge. While this system may work to enhance some professions, and some professionals and technicians, it is far from satisfactory for all as it leaves a great deal to be desired in providing integrated service delivery for the consumer.

We are faced, therefore, with the need to develop educational models and a health care system which can deal with these limitations within our knowledge base and our structure of service development and delivery. The problem is a vastly complex one with deep roots in theory limitation, and with technical and practical problems of operation. Perhaps the most complex aspect of all is the difficulty we have in changing a system practiced a long time and in which we have a deep personal, professional, and technical investment.

EDUCATIONAL PROGRAM PLANNING

Educators need to develop educational models to fit the service systems evolving in response to the broader goals of health and rehabilitation. These educational strategies are attempting to: 1) assess the tasks to be accomplished or problems to be solved; 2) determine type or level of skill and knowledge needed for each problem area; 3) plan appropriate curricula and programs for the tasks involved and the skill or knowledge level required; 4) plan within the cultural, social and economic context of the group or society involved.

These generic or universal requirements need to be met, whether planning is done for a specialized cultural group within a society or for a larger unit such as a state or country. A professional educational plan to meet health and rehabilitation needs on the Sioux Rosebud Indian Reservation will possess generic similarities, but will be different from a plan for a program in a large urban area of New York State. The tools, techniques, methods and concepts may be universal but can only be useful when adapted to the social and cultural group involved. Lifestyles, value patterns, technical, social, and educational developments, and economic resources are among areas needing consideration in any educational planning.[12]

Educational programs of the past have provided sufficient focus on interdisciplinary curricula. There is a tendency on the part of educators to believe that a curriculum is changed by adding new knowledge or new approaches. A major task must also be to weed out what is irrelevant. Such a philosophy can also be transferred into an effective service system.

First, an awareness must be created that the educational process for the health and helping professions is not now designed to satisfy the full spectrum of health maintenance. Then, the need for a clearer delineation of the interdependence of responsibility and performance among providers will become evident. Common bases of knowledge and skills shared by all health and helping professionals can be identified at each level of expertise, distinguishing those knowledges and skills that are unique and of current need from those that are obsolete.

Fendall (1972)[13] indicated that in developing nations, "With rising standards of education, the trend is toward multipurpose workers in fewer categories with broader areas of work." Such a parsimony of professions with generic education is a desirable alternative to the proliferation of "specialists." But, even with multipurpose workers, a plan for interprofessional collaboration of such specialties is required. It is difficult, and some think impossible once a specialty has been created, to combine it with another, rearrange its tasks or roles, or eliminate it totally. Personal and group identification and investment are hard to redirect and can only be accomplished with the involvement and cooperation of the personnel involved.

Lack of acceptance of support personnel by the established professions is one of the great obstacles to their use and development. For example, the findings of Muthard and Salomone (1969) indicated that rehabilitation counselors were reluctant to share any but routine, repetitive job tasks with support personnel.[14] Understanding the contribution of each other to the total human service system is essential to gaining the perspective that individual work with consumers will not be threatened but rather enhanced and extended in its effectiveness by collaboration.

Barriers between and within the health and helping professions, associations, and agencies need to be broken down. The relationship of each profession to each other must be considered—with the starting point of discussion not based upon the relationship of the professions but rather the relationship of each to the total systems of care and the function of each in relationship to the consumer. As Fenninger (1967) stated, "Recognition of the fact that all health services exist because people *need* them, not for the convenience of those who *render* them, and generosity of one group toward another, are essential if we are to develop adequate health care for all those who need it."[15]

We are convinced that teamwork and interdisciplinary action among and between the health and helping professions will emerge if the emphasis upon our individual professionalism is underemphasized in deference to the higher goals of the entire team. In such teamwork, we will begin to understand the diversity of function that created our individual professions, and finally gain respect for that diversity. We are further convinced that as all personnel learn to work together in joint problem solving with the consumer, the new service systems will be characterized by a recognition for the participatory dignity of all.

Mary E. Switzer (1967) summarized it well: "Some authorities believe and I share their view . . . that health workers of the future, working as a unit, will care for the patient, with each member responsible for certain phases of treatment and rehabilitation, and with a sense of unity among the team members which removes the barriers of disciplinary parochialism on behalf of the patient. When this picture of practice materializes as a general pattern, we will finally see a continuous flow of expert attention to prevention, detection and diagnosis, acute care, and rehabilitation . . . all as different facets of the same process."[16]

MULTIDISCIPLINARY TEAM TRAINING

Team practice, though long considered basic to comprehensive rehabilitation, has been neglected in training and educational programs and in research. Authors have written extensively about teams but primarily in a descriptive way. Little research effort has been put forth to evaluate the work of teams. Most authors have both urged improvement of team practice and lauded teamwork, claiming that it "is the best model yet constructed for working with clients as total persons with multiple needs."[17]

After a thorough review of the literature, Wagner, (1972) concludes that successful team practice focuses on specific tasks related to consumer problems and total needs of the consumer, and unsuccessful teamwork responds to multiple tasks relating to agency or institutional decisions, role differentiation, status problems, professionalization, and protection of one's area or discipline.[18] Wagner states that the study of multidisciplinary team performance is important and of immediate concern in light of the widespread emphasis on team practice in the human services.

In the meantime, however, team practice will proceed on face validity and on the pragmatic observations and conclusions of educators and practitioners who argue against fragmentation and claim that "no treatment is medical, social, psychological, or vocational—all treatment is total."[19] Individual skill in one's own profession cannot circumvent the necessity for group skills aimed toward understanding the needs and dynamics of individuals and/problems of decision making. "Multiple leadership," Jones claims, "is an essential goal which coordinated services must set for themselves."[20]

Specific focus, then, on the theory and practice of group process is needed in education and training curricula. The development of communication, decision-making and problem-solving skills can emerge only with experiential learning and practice.

The following assumptions are considered basic to productive multidisciplinary team practice and inherent in the development of educational programs of training:

1) Specific training will help individuals operate as members of multidisciplinary teams;

2) Team training will improve members' ability to focus on and solve specific consumer problems;

3) The solutions to complex human problems are not within the province of one discipline area of service, agency, or institution;

4) The consumer should be considered a member of the team in reaching solutions to his specific problems;

5) A broader knowledge of the role of different professionals will facilitate multidisciplinary team functioning;

6) Acceptance of an extended definition and concept base
for professional role will include awareness and concern for
the consumer as a complete person;

7) Acceptance of a responsibility to relate to the consumer
on a person-to-person basis, not just in a professional area,
will involve concern for his total needs in a time of illness,
trouble or disability;

8) Willingness to initiate new and sometimes unconventional activity in the consumer's behalf will help to bridge gaps
caused by professional specialization, agency, and institutional structure.

With these assumptions in mind, a number of generic components of knowledge are needed by all team members regardless of their professional identity. We have neglected
these interfaces which bind us together in our attempts to be
unique in our roles. Education and training of new professionals should be concerned with building a common base so
that learning can proceed at three levels: (a) individual and
personal development, (b) group and social development,
and (c) specific discipline and professional knowledge, skill or
technique.

The first two have often been neglected in educational
programs and settings and the third perhaps overempha-
sized. To accomplish education and training at these three
levels requires the blending of the behavioral and social sciences with the physical sciences, and, therefore, the collaboration of these faculties in academic and clinical training.

A description of two experimental programs carried out at
the State University of New York at Buffalo will show how
multidisciplinary team training evolved through various
phases of planning and demonstration. They are 1) A Core
City Team Training Project extending over three eight-week
summer periods, and 2) A Multidiscipline Team Communication course.

The Rehabilitation Counseling Program at State University
of New York at Buffalo embarked on a pilot Core City project
during the summer of 1969. The Project's Phase II program

was carried out during the summer of 1970. The goal of the project was to discover how rehabilitation counselors could be educated and trained to become a part of the systematic solution of the problems facing the inner city.

Goals of the 1970 Phase II incorporated the results of the first summer's project and specifically planned to (a) provide students experience with multiple service delivery systems for the core city, working with multiprofessionals from other disciplines; utilizing support personnel, out-reach efforts, and other non-traditional counseling models such as advocacy and consultation; (b) develop contact with and knowledge and understanding of the resources of the community in depth; (c) gain knowledge and understanding of the nature of ghetto culture and the lifestyles of its people; (d) improve the ability of the traditional trained counselors to communicate with each other and with disadvantaged persons, non-middle class clients.

Training counselors to work with inner city problems was complicated by the noticeable lack of multidisciplinary communication in the service delivery systems for the core city. Our notion is that the person who eventually delivers help to a client, whether that helper be a rehabilitation counselor, occupational therapist or other worker, must in his training develop knowledge of other professions and knowledge of the culture and social conditions from which the clients come. Consequently, Phase III, 1971, of the Core City Program was carried out with the objective of training multiprofessionals to prepare together the health care work they would be doing in the inner city.

A group of 14 black and white students in the Rehabilitation Counseling, Nursing, Occupational Therapy, and Physical Therapy professions participated in the eight-week training program. Five additional trainees were black residents of the ghetto who were called "community needs experts." These trainees were college graduates but not associated with any particular profession.

Students were placed in rehabilitation settings for two days a week practicum, and participated in multi-learning experiences at the university. These involved:

1) Didactic Seminars—included lectures on the principles of Rehabilitation Counseling, Occupational Therapy, Physical Therapy, and Nursing; role playing exercises where students played the role of the helper, the client, or a member of the client's family; films or verbal presentations oriented toward understanding life in the ghetto; and presentations on the multi-problem families of Buffalo, and how and why they are often not helped in the absence of integrated team service.

2) Resource Seminars—took the form of weekly visits to agencies which give service to multi-problem clients from the ghetto; these provided students with knowledge of resources used to solve problems.

3) Briefing with Consultants—the students met weekly with a panel of five regular consultants, one each from Occupational Therapy, Physical Therapy, Nursing, and Rehabilitation Counseling; all five were members of the university faculty or staff. Students were asked to use the knowledge and skills of the consultants for solving problems they encounter in clinical centers.

4) Skill Training Seminars—were weekly sessions designed to teach interpersonal communication skills. These sessions were exercises in basic counseling skills; students learned to discriminate and demonstrate levels of empathy, congruence, and positive regard.

5) Process Group Experience—trainees met weekly to share and discuss feelings with the objective of developing self-awareness and sensitivity to the feelings and behavior of others.

6) Practicum—students were placed in a rehabilitation facility two days a week; their job was to work with two to five disadvantaged black clients who were disabled. The placements included the Veterans Administration Hospital, Children's Hospital Rehabilitation Center, West Seneca State School for the Retarded, Booth Memorial Hospital, Talbert Mall Clinic, and Buffalo Goodwill Industries—a group of agencies with diverse and multi-problem families.

An evaluation of the summer project concluded that students who participated in the summer training were more knowledgeable of the roles and functions of other professions than students who did not and were more aware of the needs and problems of ghetto residents. Students of all disciplines began to see themselves as resource persons for the client. Regular consultations and experience with members of other professions broadened the scope in which students saw their own professions. All students became more concerned about the importance of being skilled in communication and perceived some level of counseling as being part of their job. Counselors as well as other students expressed heightened concern for diet, living conditions, and community problems.

MULTIDISCIPLINARY TEAM COMMUNICATION COURSE

Results of these three summer projects suggested that special training and experience in the interpersonal communication process for students of the health and helping professions would improve health care delivery and prepare students to function more effectively on a team in a clinical setting. Implicit was the mandate that some kind of multidisciplinary experience needs to be offered students being trained in the various professional schools.

The multidisciplinary team communication course was initiated as a joint project of the Rehabilitation Counseling Program and the School of Health Related Professions in the fall of 1971. Faculty from the Rehabilitation Counseling Program, Occupational Therapy, Physical Therapy, Speech Pathology, Nursing, and Medicine programs met and developed a course plan implementing the following objectives: 1) To offer students increased awareness and appreciation of multidisciplinary colleagues; 2) To provide students with knowledge of concepts and principles of health care personnel; 3) To transfer this knowledge and understanding of multidisciplinary teams to actual practice by functioning together as a multipersonal clinical team; 4) To create in the student a deeper awareness and understanding of emotions, attitudes, values and ideals which influence the development of service systems.

These objectives are currently being implemented in the multidisciplinary team communication course, a "demonstration" course approved by the curriculum committee of the university. Advanced students and faculty of the six programs mentioned met for three hours a week during the fourteen-week semester to work as a team, sharing the problems and experience of their agency or hospital work and using each other for resource and guidance. Students and faculty alike developed a new appreciation of other disciplines in health care.

A number of other multidisciplinary training projects are in various stages of development at the State University of New York at Buffalo. Each will serve in the future as concrete attempts to develop models of multidisciplinary team relationships in which consumers, students, and faculty plan, implement, and evaluate as the basis for future programs. Frustration with artificial barriers in the form of administrative structure and past practice in both the university and larger community is often experienced and must be overcome to bring concrete plans to fruition.

The other projects underway and their training objectives are:

Rural Health Manpower: Externship Project. Training objective: This program, in its third year of operation, provides students in the fields of medicine, dentistry, nursing, rehabilitation counseling, pharmacy, and allied health areas with summer experience in rural primary health care settings in the lower tier counties of Western New York State.

Interdisciplinary Training in Community Health (ITCH). Training objective: This project proposes to provide a setting in which ghetto community-university cooperation will lead to new opportunities to develop interdisciplinary training modalities. Clinical interdisciplinary team educational programs will be centered at two community health centers in the inner city.

Consortium for Allied Health: Disadvantaged Students. Training objective: Through the joint efforts of many of the health and helping professions on this campus, this project's goal is to organize a regional consortium of the allied health training programs in Western New York, including representatives from university, college, community college, urban centers, and hospital programs. A special emphasis will be placed on the identification, recruitment, and preparation of minority students (black, Spanish-surname, and American Indian) for careers in allied health and helping fields.

Interdisciplinary Team Experience in Extended Care Facilities and Nursing Homes. Training objective: This project will propose to explore interdisciplinary team relationships in facilities for the geriatric populations, both well and disabled. Effective utilization of health and helping personnel will seek to replace custodial care practices with rehabilitative services, including out-patient and ambulatory care programs.

In addition to these projects, consideration is underway for the planning and implementation of multidisciplinary rehabilitation potential in correctional institutions and family practice clinics with out-reach opportunities in the home and community. The ultimate goal is to formulate as a regular part of the curriculum, a team training program for all students, based on what is being learned and experienced in these projects. In addition, university faculty and staff should be available to consult with community teams and help develop and improve multidiscipline team functioning.

We are convinced that the expansion of comprehensive health care and rehabilitation services into many *new* clinical centers will assure unique and expanding roles for allied health and the helping professions. Neighborhood health care centers and multi-purpose centers, nursing homes and extended care facilities, rehabilitation centers for multi-problems, half-way houses, transitional housing services, workshops and work evaluation programs, inner-city health projects, and rural health manpower resources—these new out-reach projects and programs, which are attempting to respond to important social and health needs—will seldom reach fruition without the availability of allied health and helping professionals to assist in planning, staffing, and evaluating these new program approaches.

Cultural Universals

There is a need to state with clarity that no program of service or training can be developed within the context of one society or culture, and be transplanted in total to another. Each program plan of education and service must be tailored and developed to the needs, value patterns, social context, and economic and manpower resources specific to that society or country.[21] However, it is also our belief that there are certain generic features or principles of the health and helping process which relate to all societies or cultures, based on our common humanity and the universality of human need. Most of these concepts have already been discussed in relation to certain topics in the context of the paper, but they are summarized for purposes of clarity.

1) Illness and disability and ways or patterns of coping with them are universal in all societies. Acceptance of dependency resulting from illness and disability is assumed by a society or culture as its economic, social, and cultural resources permit. The plans of care are in keeping with the value patterns and available resources within that society or culture.

2) The holistic nature of man is universal in all societies. To divide people and services into parts such as medical, social, psychological, and educational, relates more to the needs and convenience of practitioners, organizations, and agencies than to the needs of consumers.

3) A generic base of education and training within the health and helping professions is essential for the development of comprehensive health maintenance and rehabilitation systems. Holist needs of consumers require a coming together of the physical, social, and psychological disciplines in the development of educational programs and service systems. Generic training will facilitate a common communication base and thus foster this multidiscipline collaboration.

4) All-purpose workers make possible a desirable parsimony in numbers of professionals and also diminish fragmentation of service. Though a desirable goal in service delivery, it must be balanced with the professional's need to deal

with the reality of ever-increasing knowledge and technology. One way of coping with this problem has been the emergence of increasing numbers of professionals and technicians.

5) Focus on group process, as a specific part of educational and training programs, will help professionals communicate and function more effectively as members of multi-disciplinary teams. Such team training will increase knowledge of different professions and improve members' ability to focus on and solve specific consumer problems, thereby diminishing service gaps and fragmentation.

6) The process of evaluating and improving service delivery to consumers should be a continuing activity focused on tasks and problems, rather than on professional roles and rights. A willingness to initiate new and often unconventional service plans or systems may be necessary in the consumer's behalf to confront gaps in service and agency or professional specialization.

7) Consumers of comprehensive services of health and rehabilitation have inherent resources within striving toward health; these resources need to be mobilized and used in fostering programs of self-help. The consumer needs to be a member of his own rehabilitation team to partake in the development and decide on plans to maintain and sustain his own physical and mental health. Services exist for consumers who need them, not for the convenience of professionals who render them.

NOTES

1. E. D. Pellegrino, "Health Maintenance: An idea in search of an organization." Distinguished Lecture in conjunction with James Fenton Lecture Series and Institute on Health Maintenance: Challenge for Allied Health Professions, State University of New York at Buffalo, School of Health Related Professions, October, 1971, p. 15 (modified and appearing as a chapter in this book).

2. M. E. Jaques, "Rehabilitation Counseling and Support Personnel," *Rehabilitation Counseling Bulletin*, Vol. 15, No. 3 (March, 1972): 160-171; J. W. Perry, "Career Mobility in Allied Health Education," *Journal of American Medical Assn.*, 210 (October 6, 1969):107-110.

3. *Alcoholics Anonymous.* Alcoholics Anonymous World Services, Inc. (New York: 1955).

4. A. A. Low, *Mental Health Through Will Training* (Boston: Christopher Publishing House, 1950).

5. D. Krech, "Does behavior really need a brain? In Praise of William James: Some historical musings, vain lamentations, and a sounding of great expectations," *William James: Unfinished Business*, ed. R. B. MacLeod (Washington, D.C.: American Psychological Assn., Inc., 1969).

6. K. Goldstein, "The Organismic Approach," *American Handbook of Psychiatry*, Vol. 2, ed. S. Arieti (New York: Basic Books, Inc., 1959).

7. A. H. Maslow, *Toward a Psychology of Being* (Princeton, N.J.: D. Van Nostrand Co., Inc., 1962).

8. F. Goble, *The Third Force, The Psychology of Abraham Maslow* (New York: Grossman Publishers, Inc., 1970. Pocket Book Edition, New York: 1971).

9. F. Perls, R. Hefferline, and P. Goodman, *Gestalt Therapy* (New York: Julian Press, Inc., 1951. Paperback, New York: Dell Publishing Co., Inc., 1965).

10. F. S. Perls, *In and Out of the Garbage Pail* (Lafayette, Calif.: Real People Press, 1969. Paperback, New York: Bantam Books, Inc., 1972).

11. M. E. Jaques, *Rehabilitation Counseling: Scope and Services* (Boston: Houghton Mifflin Company, 1970).

12. C. Safilios-Rothschild, *The Sociology and Social Psychology of Disability and Rehabilitation* (New York: Random House, 1970).

13. N. R. E. Fendall, *Auxiliaries in Health Care: Programs in Developing Countries* (Baltimore: The Johns Hopkins Press, 1972), p. 14.

14. J. E. Muthard and R. R. Salomone, "Roles and Functions of the Rehabilitation Counselor," *Rehabilitation Counseling Bulletin*, Special Issue, 13, (1-SP), October, 1969.

15. L. Fenninger, "The Allied Health Professions—at the Flood Tide of Opportunity." Manpower Conference for the Health Related Professions.

16. M. E. Switzer, "Serving is a privilege, not a problem," Manpower Conference for the Health Related Professions, State University of New York at Buffalo, 1967.

17. M. E. Jaques, *Rehabilitation Counseling*, p. 7.

18. R. J. Wagner, "A Comparison of the Performance of Multidisciplinary Teams and Independent Practitioners." Unpublished doctoral dissertation in process, Rehabilitation Counseling Program, State University of New York at Buffalo, 1972. York, 1972.

19. F. A. Whitehouse, "Teamwork: A Democracy of Professions." *Exceptional Children* 18 (46) (November, 1951):45-52.

20. M. Jones, *Beyond the Therapeutic Community: Social Learning and Social Psychiatry* (New Haven: Yale University Press, 1968), p. 37.

21. "The development of rehabilitation services in relation to available resources," *Rehabilitation International, Technical Paper No. 23* (New York: International Society for Rehabilitation of the Disabled, 1969).

HEALTH CARE &
THE HEALTH MARKET

Samuel P. Martin

Health and medical care, catapulted from its mystic, semi-religious ethos into the middle of the modern industrial world, is now America's third largest industry.[1] Between 1950 and 1970 the health-related labor force increased 83 percent while the general labor force increased only 22 percent.[2] In 1972 the health and medical care industry spent a sum of money greater than 7 percent of the gross national product, nearly twice the proportionate amount spent by other industrial countries.[3]

America has a per capita spending for health and medical care greater than any other country and more physicians per capita than any country except Israel.[4] Despite all these glowing statistics, however, the system provided fewer office visits per person in 1968 than in 1958 and no dramatic shift in morbidity or mortality rates; in fact, death rates rose in that decade.[5]

This massive spending and the results bring up some serious questions: Are we getting the greatest possible benefit from our expenditure? Is our expenditure being used most effectively?

The application of economic techniques to the health field is not new. In a recent historical review of this development, Rashi Fein points out that economic analyses of the value of human life were begun in the latter part of the seventeenth century by physicians to justify governmental expenditure for health and sanitation programs.[6] Sir William Petty, an anatomist, placed a value of 69 to 90 pounds sterling on man, deriving his figures from the productive contribution of man's labor. He also calculated the loss to England from "plague, slaughter of men in war, and sending troops abroad in the services of foreign princes."

Chadwick, in the mid-1800s, made useful economic estimates on loss caused by excessive sickness, premature disability, and death. He described programs of sanitation as "an economic question of production," pleading that in addition to sustaining a humane view of man, we should adopt a systematic economic view of man as an investment in capital in a productive labor force.

In America, Lemuel Shattuck viewed sanitary programs in light of their potential yield and calculated the loss to Massachusetts caused by failure to institute public health measures. Farr refined the techniques to estimate the economic worth of man. In a recent classic monograph describing the losses from various disease entities, Dorothy Rice points out the total costs of disease by systems, and estimates the economic loss from illness, disability, and death in 1963 to be in the range of 105 billion dollars.[7]

While most past data have dealt with macroeconomics, there has been a recent movement into consideration of the specific cost of programs, cost of production, and benefit —that is, into *microeconomics*. Gill defines microeconomics as "the way in which individual units that make up the economy—private consumer, business firms, laborers, landowners, producers of particular commodities or services—act and react upon each other and in their interaction meet many of society's needs. This field is contrasted with macroeconomics, which considers broad social aggregates like national income, total employment, inflation, and the growth of output over time."[8]

THE MEDICAL-HEALTH CARE MARKET

This paper will review some aspects of the medical-health care market. Figure 1 is a schematic representation of the industrial market, taken from an article by Fuchs,[9] showing the firm, the producer, and the household—that is, the con-

Figure 1

Model of the Market (Fuchs)

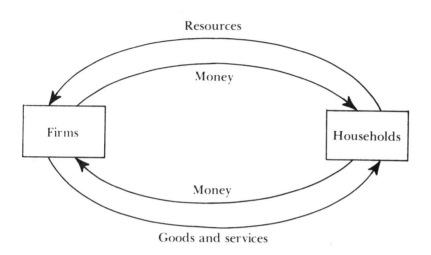

sumer. Figure 2 is an adaptation of Figure 1 designed to illustrate the medical-health care market. The household provides the resources, and the firm converts them into a product. Money is the mode of exchange. In this exchange, the "invisible hand of the market," in the words of Adam Smith, regulates "the what" "the how," and "the to whom." The equation of this market may be expressed as follows:

Equation 1 (Market)

CD + CA = Demand = Supply = PA + PD

CD = Consumer Demand

CA = Consumer Ability

PA = Producer Ability

PD = Producer Desire

The special nature of the medical-health care market introduces a number of problems in defining its parts (Figure 2). The medical firm has elements of its semireligious ethos and its paternalism existing side by side with its modern industrial ethos. Some groups, such as hospital administrators, have tried to rationalize the firm in terms of modern industrial ethos, but find it difficult. The firm may be defined as the

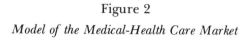

Figure 2

Model of the Medical-Health Care Market

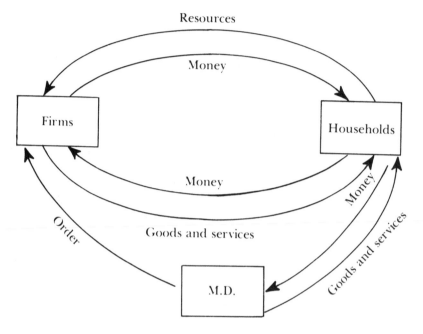

whole medical core industry, which would include offices, hospitals, clinics, drug firms, and laboratories. One economist has viewed the home as the firm in that the object of the firm is to produce health, not to treat illness.[10]

The location of the physician in the diagram is difficult. He eschews the position of member of the firm; thus we have the system of dual authority prevalent in many hospitals, clinics, and laboratories.[11] Some look at him as a salesman for the firm. Kenneth Arrow views him as a trustee for the consumer; in this capacity, he would remain outside the household, but be related to it.[12]

Among the unusual characteristics of the medical-health care markets is a problem of product uncertainty: Is the product maintenance of health, or is it treatment of disease? This duality makes demand rather peculiar. If the product is maintenance of health, then demand is universal, predictable, and evenly distributed, for the product is desirable as well as satisfying. If, however, the product is treatment of illness, then demand is non-universal, unpredictable, and non-random in its distribution, for the product is needed only when the client is in an abnormal state. Consumption and subsequent satisfaction are hard to characterize because of the natural healing capacity of the body. Moreover, many modalities of treatment, quite successful and popular in the past, have been found later to have no benefit.

Then, entry into the market has a number of special strictures. The number of places where the doctor may be trained is severely limited by the high cost of medical education, which in turn is related to the standards set by the profession and monitored by accreditation bodies. Accreditation rules are not open to public influence, but are set by educators. Licensure may to some extent limit entry in states that require special qualifications, such as citizenship. Certification, which is used in addition to licensure in many health-related professions, is another restrictive factor. In medicine, board certification has been used by some hospitals to determine staff appointments and compensation.

Entrepreneurship and prices are also restricted in the medical-health care market. Price discrimination has existed for years under the guise of lower prices for the lower-income groups. Elaborate relative value codes for procedures have been worked out and conversion factors have been negotiated to control floor prices. Although not mandatory, such a system could not operate in other markets without legal action on the grounds of price-fixing. Many states have legal restrictions against corporate practice and advertising. Medical societies have stringent rules covering marketing.

Another unusual characteristic lies in the two types of inputs seen in the package of care: physicians' services, and products and technical services. There are serious production constraints on physicians' services and no constraints on products and technical services. The situation is not unlike the abnormal state of the automobile industry after World War II, when cars were hard to obtain, but accessories were readily available. The dealer could sell stripped down models, or those with every available accessory; he tended to try to do the latter.

Lastly, the medical-health care market has the problem of self-generation of demand by the firm, a problem that will be reviewed throughout the remainder of this presentation. With such an array of distorting features as has been indicated for it, it is not surprising that economists say that the "invisible hand" in the medical-health care market is "all thumbs."

To try to picture the market in a manner similar to Equation 1, requires two equations rather than one:

Equation 2 (Medical-Health Care Market):
Equation 2A:
   CD + CA = Initial Visit = Rq
   Rq = Requisition for care

In this equation, the consumer decides that he will enter the market and, on entering, the physician assumes control. He produces services and requests others.

Equation 2B:
   CA + Rq + PD = Demand = Supply = AHC + DHC
   PD = Physician Demand
   AHC = Ability of Health Care System
   DHC = Desire of Health Care System

Equation 2A is client-centered. Its rate is dependent on the client and the availability of services. Whether or not one individual seeks medical care depends on his psychological make-up, his culture, his education, and his financial ability, in about that order. Suchman points out that only eight percent of a sample indicated financial concern in seeking care.[13] For psychological reasons, many people do not perceive symptoms as abnormal or needing attention. In many cultures, care is not sought because to do so seems an indication of weakness. If the patient decides to act, he must find an available portal to enter care. Sometimes its location is obscure to him, or the queue is long. Also, many physicians will not accept new patients.

Equation 2B is physician-centered. After the client makes the requisition, the physician's demands far outweigh the client's influence. The physician is quick to give examples of the client demand for antibiotics or other treatment, as well as the threat of malpractice; however, these pressures play a minor role and are open to modulation by the physician. Demand on the part of the physician, like that coming from the client, depends on his psychological make-up, his culture, his education, and his financial need. Again, the importance is about the same as the order in which they are listed. From the psychological perspective, the self-confidence of the physician can regulate the extent to which he uses tests to confirm his clinical impressions; some physicians are compulsive.

As for cultural regulation, the Joint Commission on Hospital Accreditation, for example, can write into its regulations the routine demand for certain services, and hospital staff regulations can require specific procedures. Looking at education, one can observe that during early medical school and residency training, many procedures used in medical care are used for the dual purpose of medical care and medical education. In the educational process, after the learning of physiological and biochemical mechanisms, there is no debriefing period that separates the care and the educational functions of various procedures. Thus, our educational system turns out a practitioner who may have mixed motives in using these procedures. Indeed, one finds many fewer procedures used in other countries of the medical-care world than ours.

Lastly, the financial needs of the physician obviously have some impact on the availability of service. Studies on hours per week of practice and change in medical care price index were presented in a review of practices in *Medical Economics:*[14] When the price index rose sharply in 1968, the hours devoted to service dropped. The physician not only controls the intensity of his work, but also the mix of his personal services with those generated by the technology. For example, addition of the multi-channel laboratory chemical analyser adds markedly to the services that can be easily mobilized, but it is difficult to bring together services requiring an input of the physician's personal time that is not open to technological expansion.

Figure 3

Supply-Demand Plot for Equation 2A and 2B Functions of Medical Care

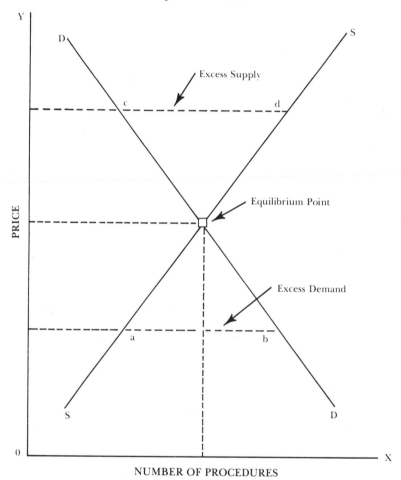

NUMBER OF PROCEDURES

Equilibrium price and quantity will be determined at the intersection of the supply-demand curves.

PRICING IN THE
MEDICAL-HEALTH CARE MARKET

Using the equation for the market, an open market such as Equation 1, we can use a diagram from Gill,[15] which has been modified to cover medical care (Figure 3). This diagram shows a supply and demand plot. Price is plotted on the Y axis and quantity on the X axis. Line SS is supply and DD is demand. On the open market, supply seeks demand and the price is reached at the equilibrium point. As supply increases, demand is satisfied—and with its satisfaction, need will drop, with a concomitant fall in price until that equilibrium point is reached.

In the medical situation, one can draw a supply-demand curve for Equation 2A and Equation 2B. Because of the external pressures on the medical-health care market described previously, the point where the market rests is not the equilibrium point. In Equation 2A, the price is low, the supply limited, and the demand great. This is represented by point *a* in Figure 3. The difference between point *a* and point *b* is the excess in demand. This would be the supply-demand-price-quantity situation for initial visits to the physician. Feldstein characterizes the medical-health care market generally at this position.[16] An office or home visit has a low price, and is hard to obtain, often occurring at the end of long waits.

In Equation 2B the supply-demand is represented by point *c*. Here the price is high; the supply is excessive. Examples would be surgical operations, or laboratory tests. There is no long wait, and it is easy to find someone who will convert the requisition into a service.

Table 1[17] shows some examples of the prices of items covered by Equation 2A and 2B. When these are presented in this fashion, it is hard to comprehend why a urinalysis is equal in price to a brief examination. The supply of urinalyses is limitless, and the cost is minimal compared with the price. Many laboratory procedures, as well as other 2B procedures, are priced at levels four to ten times the cost. Tonsillectomies with or without adenoidectomies are priced at three times the value of initial comprehensive history and physical examina-

Table 1

Medical Prices

Taken from Massachusetts Relative Value Scale and Conversion
Factor as of October 1972.[17]

Procedure	*Equation 11A Functions*
Initial limited history and physical examination including initiation of diagnostic and treatment program	$15.00
Initial comprehensive history and physical examination including initiation of diagnosis and treatment program	35.00
Established patient minimal service	4.00
Brief examination evaluation and/or treatment of same or new illness	6.00
Home visit, initial limited visit	20.00
Equation 11B Functions	
Tonsillectomy with or without adenoidectomy under age 12	100.00
Total hysterectomy (corpus & cervix)	400.00
Urinalysis routine complete	6.00
PO_2, PCO_2 and pH arterial blood	50.00
Aldosterone urine, double isotope dilution	120.00
Bone marrow aspiration and interpretation	35.00
Autopsy examination including CNS gross & microscopic	360.00

tion, including initiation of a diagnosis and treatment program. In tonsillectomy, this price does not include the hospital overhead required to perform the procedure. Total hysterectomy (without hospital overhead) is over ten times the price of an initial examination.

When one looks at the capacity of the system to produce and the apparent need, one finds most Equation 2B functions to be at point c in the area of excess supply. How can either the situation of point a or point c exist? In other markets, such situations have existed only under governmental control, monopoly, or restricted competition. The abnormality of the medical-health care market supports this disequilibrium. The laws of supply and demand are not inviolable, but generally, under any condition, it is difficult to support indefinitely a skewed system. Even under governmental price fixing, a black market will develop.

THREE TASKS

There are three tasks an economic system must perform:[18] 1) it must allocate the efforts of society to production of the goods and services needed by that society; 2) it must determine the methods of production; and 3) it must solve the problem of distributing the output among its members. These tasks correspond to the "what," the "to whom," and the "how" of the medical market.

THE "WHAT" OF THE
MEDICAL-HEALTH CARE MARKET

The "what" of the medical-health care market is the kinds of health care goods and services to be produced. There are a number of ways these can be divided. One would involve the split between primary, secondary, and tertiary care functions. Emphasis in the recent past has obviously been placed on secondary and tertiary care. In 1929 to 1931, the Committee on Cost of Medical Care found 62.8 percent of the people in a statistical sample availed themselves of medical care in a twelve-month period.[19] The Committee's sample was composed of white families. In 1958 the National Opinion Research Survey showed 66 percent of its sample visited a physician.[20]

According to estimates from the Health Interview Survey, conducted by the National Center for Health Statistics, there were 927 million physician visits in the United States in 1970 (including telephone contacts), an average of 4.6 per person.[21] Seventy-two percent of the population consulted a physician at least once that year, the survey showed. The shift is manifested not only by the increasing specialization of physicians, but also by the growth of the subspecialties and the emphasis on hospitalization while primary care physicians are decreasing. During this interval, biomedical research has stressed basic biological mechanisms and their application to severe illness. There has been little research into determination of vulnerability, early detection of disease, or early intervention techniques.

Another division would be between the care and the cure functions of the industry. The cure function is highly favored, as manifested by our massive efforts in cancer therapy and cardiac surgery, but efforts supporting the care function have been limited. The care of the incurable takes second place in our society, and palliation is low on the therapeutic approach. Instead, radical and fruitless procedures are frequently attempted. Also, the client is not always brought face-to-face with the decision-making process. With data, the patient might choose a different course.

In either case, as will be highlighted later, we tend to give what can be expanded easily, like the functions of Equation 2B such as laboratory tests, rather than find ways to expand the functions of Equation 2A such as visits to the medical care establishment.

THE "TO WHOM" OF THE
MEDICAL-HEALTH CARE MARKET

In most American enterprise, particularly the product industries, the "to whom" is left to the "invisible hand" of the market. Mass production, installment buying, mass merchandising, and competitive entrepreneurship have made televisions and clothes washers household items in many, many homes. In other American enterprises, particularly the service industries, government agencies have regulated not only quality of service and price, but also distribution—for example, in banking, utilities, and transportation. Thus, to receive a franchise, a utility frequently has to serve a geographic area with both high and low profit centers.

Hart has stated that in the health service industry there is an

"Inverse Care Law": Briefly, the availability of good medical care tends to vary inversely with the need of the population served.[22] A study of a county in Indiana in 1929[23] and a view of the same county today demonstrates the trend toward centralization of services. In 1929, physicians were distributed in many parts of the county, but now they are concentrated in certain areas, and many outlying communities are without physicians.

THE "HOW" OF THE
MEDICAL-HEALTH CARE MARKET

The producer in the product industry (Equation 1) is acutely aware of the economics of production. He can tell to the tenths and hundredths of a cent the cost of production, and is always alert to means of altering production by use of less expensive material, mechanization, reorganization, and other factors to deliver the product to the buyer at the lowest cost consistent with quality and a profit. Parts of a cent may mean survival. Sometimes he cuts the price a little too sharply, with disastrous effects for himself or the consumer or both. The "how" of production involves the methods whereby the goods and services are put together to form a product. What goes into production? Here the producer and society must weigh effectiveness of production and benefit to society. In the "how" of the market, there is a fine balance between effective production, and delivering a poor product.

A producer in the industrial world is acutely aware of the cost centers. He knows where the costs of production come from, and can give attention to the more expensive elements. In many offices, clinics, and hospitals we have little knowledge of any cost other than total cost. We do not know the cost of a specific procedure, test, or service.

Figure 4 represents hypothetical cost-production curves for three diseases. On the X axis is plotted the health achieved or illness eliminated, and on the Y axis is plotted the money expended (cost). The three diseases are acute appendicitis, acute lobar pneumonia, and myocardial infarct. For the purpose of discussion, the mortality-morbidity would be assumed

52

Figure 4

Three Hypothetical Curves of Cost-Health Interrelation

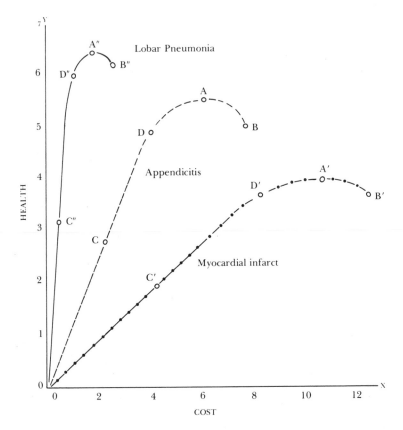

to be high if the diseases are untreated. As more services are given, the health achieved will increase and mortality-morbidity will fall off.

The rate of decline depends on the nature of the disease, and inputs in service. In appendectomy, a kitchen table removal might be equivalent to point C on the curve. Removal on an ambulant basis in a modern operating room and return home may be point D, and four days in a hospital may be point A. Point B would represent all accomplished at point A, plus intestinal moniliasis from unnecessary antibiotic therapy.

As the first or basic inputs are applied, the health achieved will increase rapidly, and mortality and morbidity will fall off sharply, but further additions will have a decreasing impact until at some point (A on curve), further expenditure will not improve health by reduction of mortality and morbidity. Increasing expenditures beyond point A will actually be associated with increased mortality or morbidity, because most of our therapeutic instruments carry a risk (point B). Limiting inputs may produce results comparable to point C or to point D. Similar curves could be developed for the other diseases. The slopes of the curves, the cost for maximal benefit, and the total benefits will vary with each disease.

Figure 5 represents the data from treatment of acute appendicitis plotted in another fashion: The gain in health is plotted on the Y axis against a unit of expenditure at each level of expenditure on the X axis. The first unit of expenditure produced an enormous drop in mortality or morbidity; this could be the kitchen table appendectomy. The second unit produced a much smaller drop; this would be the addition of a modern hospital operating room. The third unit would produce less, and so on until point A on Figure 3 is reached. Further addition of procedures, techniques, or drugs would only produce complications and decrease health with increased morbidity and mortalities. One notes that the expenditure increases more rapidly than the impact on mortality and morbidity as one approaches the A points on the three curves. The change in morbidity-mortality decreases with cost. The difference between the D points and the A points on the curve is small for the difference in expenditure, and introduces the question of the value of the increased expenditure.

In order to approach some of these problems, we undertook a view change in medical-health care for a series of diseases over the last thirty years. These studies were done by Mr. Charles Wisseman at the University of Pennsylvania, a freshman medical student, and Drs. Donaldson and London, senior students at Harvard.

Two voluntary community hospitals were used. Excellent medical records were readily available for the previous thirty years. (The hospitals have limited house-staff programs.) Patient records were collected consecutively for an entire year,

Figure 5

*Amount of Health or Illness Produced by a Unit
of Expenditure at Various Levels of Expenditure*

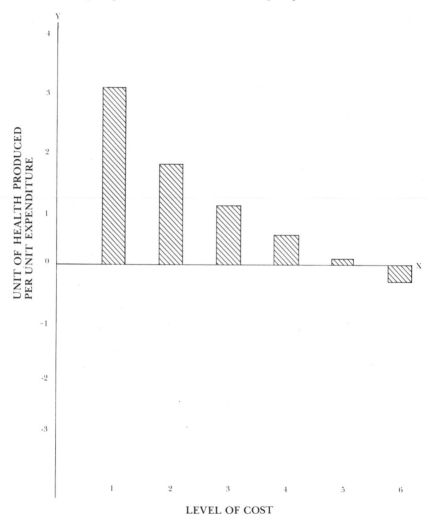

and the years were selected to give the widest possible variation in cost and pattern of treatment; i.e., pre-World War II to present. All procedures, tests, and medications were tabulated. The patients were classified by disease severity. In the case of acute appendicitis, the patients were divided into two groups: those having simple appendicitis, and those having perforation with peritonitis. The age and sex distributions in 1939 and 1969 were the same.

The inputs into care such as blood counts, chemistries, and x-rays showed 10- to 100-fold increases. The days in the hospital during this interval, however, showed significant decrease, and the mortality dropped from 5 and 33 percent to zero. In contrast, with myocardial infarction the inputs showed as much as a 200-fold increase, with *no* change in duration of hospitalization. There was a decrease in mortality between 1939 and 1949, but no marked change thereafter. In the group with appendicitis, the mortality and morbidity decreased during the period.

We need to know which of the inputs was associated with the improved outcome. Was it the added tests, the added people in the operating room, or the antibiotic medication? With myocardial infarction, there was no change in morbidity and no recent change in mortality. Are the increased inputs justified? It becomes important to sort out the productive and non-productive inputs.

Studies on ambulant surgery or early discharge are being conducted in various parts of the world, and may isolate the important factor or factors. Some studies indicate, for example, that patients discharged one day after surgery do as well as those discharged in the above series on the eighth day.[24]

While our studies of myocardial infarction were being done, a controlled clinical study was completed by Mather and his colleagues in England.[25] Individuals were randomly assigned to home and inpatient care. They could show no impact of hospitalization on outcome. This result raised questions about hospitalization for the mild myocardial infarctions. Studies by Harpur and colleagues showed that patients could be discharged on the fifteenth day and return to work on the thirtieth, without adverse effect on mortality or complication rates.[26] If this routine had been applied to the mycocardial infarction series, it would have saved twelve hospital days. Review of the production function brings into sharp focus not only the concept of marginal productivity, but also the importance of searching for the point of maximum benefit and the most effective production method.

In another study, Bloom and others applied economic techniques to the evaluation of x-ray therapy units.[27] They made no effort to quantitate output beyond cases treated. The study covered units in a wide geographic area, divided into two groups: high-usage and low-usage, both dealing with the same case mix. In the high-usage group, there was a 30 percent difference in the unit cost of treatment. Within the low-usage group, there was a 275 percent difference between the highest and lowest usage. This difference points to a wide variation in the effectiveness of the units. The high-usage units treated mostly neoplastic diseases, while the low-usage units treated many non-neoplastic diseases.

Bloom and Peterson have also studied coronary care units, finding here, also, wide variations in cost, in utilization by patients with infarction, and in mortality. If such wide differences existed in the industrial world, for example in the auto or appliance industry, they would end in bankruptcy for the less effective, more costly units.

MARGINAL UTILITY AND THE
MEDICAL-HEALTH CARE MARKET

One of the great discoveries in economics is the concept of marginal utility. With the examples of ineffective, nonproductive inputs and the concept of overkill in medicine, it is obvious that this concept has not pervaded the production system of medical and health care. The marginal utility of a commodity has been defined by Gill as the addition to our total ability (or satisfaction) occasioned by the last unit of the commodity in our possession.[28] This concept can be applied to the individual patient or to the group.

The first situation, the individual, is presented in Figure 4. For an individual with myocardial infarct, there is little gain from expenditure between point D and point A. The difference between these two points could, for example, represent the difference between discharge on the fifteenth and the twenty-eighth day. This difference could amount to as much as a thousand dollars. If the patient with proper knowledge could choose between spending the thousand dollars on staying in the hospital or spending the money on a new car, a few sessions of marriage counseling, an elevator in his home, or a short course in his business or professional area, a significant number might feel that any of these could help him return to a productive life better than continuing a hospital stay.

There is a question of marginal utility for society as well as for the client. This is a difficult issue for the physician, since his traditional orientation is to the individual—his patient —rather than society; that is, he has tended to give his patient everything regardless of others. When the total toll reaches a certain point, however, history has shown a consumer shift.

Figure 6 shows a marginal utility curve modified for medical care.[29] On the Y axis is plotted the marginal utility in units of satisfaction, and on the X axis is plotted number of surgical operations (hysterectomies) per 10,000 hospital discharges. Along the line M-M are placed the points for New England (A), Liverpool (B), and Upsala (C).[30]

As the number of operations is increased, the satisfaction given society by further increase is less than the satisfaction society might obtain if the money were spent in other areas. When the patients with tumors of such size and nature as to warrant removal have been operated upon, and the severe prolapses have been corrected, the need for operation begins to diminish and the operations done for less severe disease are less rewarding to the society. It would be interesting to have a clear idea of the point where this finding begins to appear. Is it at levels higher than those of the U.S., or is it nearer to the English or Swedish experience? Clearly, as one approaches pricing and allocation of resources in the medical market for vast numbers of procedures covered by Equation 2B, this must be determined.

Utilizing the concept of marginal utility to help in the process of allocation of limited resources has been developed to a

high degree. In the defense area, a model for such allocation has been used. In medicine, we are ready for such models for allocating resources on the basis of effectiveness, and for the benefit of programs.[31] In health, there are a number of reviews for specific programs; an example is the renal dialysis program.[32]

NON-PHYSICIAN MANPOWER AND THE MEDICAL-HEALTH CARE MARKET

There are few definitive analyses of all the possible roles the nonphysician health worker might play in the delivery of health care services. In a completely open market as visualized by economists of the free market type, anyone might set up a practice to give medical care. The practitioner would be free of all restrictions such as education, certification and licensure. The danger here is obvious. Some of these types of practitioner exist in the religious and cult healers. This system could only work with highly knowledgeable clients.

Other economists advocate a less radical approach which would involve placing practice in the hands of a corporation which would be licensed and would select its professional staff as well as assume responsibility to the client. This would substitute institutional licensure for individual licensure. The institution would thus be responsible to the public and the individual for quality of care. The corporate practice of medicine is forbidden in many states and has been vigorously opposed by the professional societies.

The present legal framework of licensure allows two kinds of roles. One is the semi-independent practitioner working under a mandate from the state or a physician with task definitions controlled by licensure or physician delegation. Another is the assistant role where each condition and situation is handled separately and on the spot. In the last hundred years in the United States, the true legal role of a wide variety of professional health workers (nonphysician) has been markedly limited by legislation but the factual role has been much less restricted. The factual role has allowed the "granny" midwife in the community, the skilled nurse in the frontier

nursing service, the psychiatric social worker in low income
community clinic. In fact, in certain disciplines such as
psychiatry, a great deal of the care of the indigent has been
given by nonphysicians.

One can only marvel at the gap between the *de facto* and
de juri functions which exist in the daily practice of medical
care. This difference is ignored by state and professional
societies until a problem develops. Problems generally come
from someone flaunting the *de facto* functions either to make
money, or to challenge the physician or the professional
societies. In some solo practice situations, one can find nurses
who may in the absence of the physician literally practice
medicine. It is interesting to speculate on the factors such as
income, accessability of manpower and care which control the
width of the gap between the *de juri* and the *de facto* state of the
nonphysician professional.

The roles of semi-independent and assistant are being tried
in an organized fashion. In both roles it becomes important to
do task analyses and job descriptions. The area of task analysis
has been developed best in dentistry and pediatrics. It has
been shown the average pediatrician spends approximately
half of his time treating well babies and a third of his time in
care of minor complaints.[33] Without task analysis, there has
been considerable confusion in finding a place for the nonphysician worker in the provision of care. A well trained
pediatric nurse practitioner may find each physician has a
different view of the tasks which should be delegated.

As a basis for delegation, some investigators advocate a split
between care and cure functions. In this system, the physician
establishes the diagnosis, writes out a medical plan, and the
allied health professional carries out the plan under supervision. The care functions have involved a great deal of a
physician's time and, on the whole, have been done poorly.

One group of investigators has advocated complete delegation of primary care to such individuals while others abhor
such delegation, stating the initial visit can be the most de-
manding and crucial part of care. Most first visits involve
self-limited minor disease processes which, if left untreated,
would resolve themselves rapidly. Hidden in this mass, how-

ever, is the patient with early obscure disease which, if detected, might have its natural course changed. The opponent
of primary care delegation finds it a paradox of thinking that
this difficult job of sorting be delegated to the least well-
trained individual. They point out, for example, that care of a
known diabetic has fewer decision-making hazards than the
determination of the significance of chest pain in a new patient who is unknown to the practice. In the former, the
problem is known and the potential for error is limited. In the
latter, the possibilities are boundless, most will be minor and
self-limited, but a rarer one will be serious.

Productivity is hard to measure in medical and health
care.[34] Simple measurements of inputs do not relate directly
to output. As noted above, output may be related to a disease
entity cured or a year free of disease. In addition to these
outputs, there are qualitative aspects of output encompassed
under such intangible terms as taste.

It is assumed that addition of allied health personnel to the
health care team will be associated with increased productivity, either their own or the physician's.

In reviewing the productivity of the allied health personnel,
one has to review their output against the cost. Since we have
so few measures of output, this is in the future. Good figures on
the cost of all allied health professionals are also needed. The
cost of education and the opportunity cost of education must
be determined and must be spread over the duration of practice of their profession. In some areas where duration of an
active career is short, it makes the total cost much higher than
the pure payroll cost. When this is done on a lifetime basis for
each health profession, it may give one a start.

Lewis and associates compared care given a sample of patients by a nurse clinic with a physician clinic.[35] There were
very significant differences in the two clinics in their pattern
of care. The nurse clinic provided more visits, less waiting,
fewer broken appointments, and less hospitalization than the
physician clinics and with very few physician consultations. It
provided a year of care at about twenty percent below the cost
of the physician clinic, much of the saving coming from decreased hospitalization. With this method of costing, a year of

care is an accurate index of productivity. While the professional salary cost of the nurse practitioner was lower by a factor of three, the patient obviously received more contacts and more time. Silver has stated that three nurse practitioners can replace the time of one pediatrician.[36] Here is an obvious potential for increased productivity and diminished cost.

This poses the ethical question of the distribution of the increased income from the increased productivity: what part should the physician be allowed to capture for himself since the physician controls the utilization of these services? In the case of products, we look with some disdain upon the physician who prescribes a product and then sells it to the client. In the example cited above by Silver, how should the pediatrician with three assistants divide the fruits of the increased productivity? Should he make the same amount as the single pediatrician or the same as two pediatricians? In pricing any product or service, it is obvious that the managers should be allowed to gain from the increased productivity. Rigid controls have inhibited technological innovation. The client should also benefit beyond more service.

In the industrial world, increased productivity frequently is converted to more income through price competition and market share. The price is lowered and in turn the added market share increases the profit; thus, both client and manager benefit. As pointed out above, such thinking does not always govern action in the medical market.

FUTURE OF THE MEDICAL-HEALTH CARE MARKET

The medical-health care market is undergoing a rapid evolution. Speculation on directions for its future would lead one to analyse the gross inconsistencies with the market and see what might happen to some of them. The most glaring inconsistency involves strictures on entrance to the market. There have been recent recommendations to increase the number of physicians.[37] This will no doubt occur, but the increase will never be sufficient to compensate for some of the other problems, such as provider-generated demand.

Another trend involves more organization of the practice

situation. Simple organization of practice into groups will not
in itself make entry more open. Yankauer found more delegation in a solo practice than in a group practice. Organization
into large groups will required a planned effort to open the
practice and patient care to the allied health professional.[38]
Group practice generally brings in helping hands but does not
change assignment of duties and definitely does not open the
market to new and new kinds of providers. With the
development of organizations such as Health Maintenance
Organizations with prepaid care, it is possible that the old
ideas and anti-industrial patterns, with their legal restrictions
on corporate practice, will be eroded as these large organizations receive a mandate to give care.

The concept of payment by capitation is introducing a new
element into the ethos of the medical-health care market.
Under fee-for-service, the patient or his third party paid the
fee and the physician's income depended on utilization by
client. Under prepayment by client and capitation payment of
the physician, increased utilization of all types could actually
increase his work without increasing his income. In fact,
under capitation, non-utilization is highly desirable for the
provider. It is possible that the opposite of over-utilization
could develop under the prepayment by client and capitation
payment of physician.

Medical foundations, also growing rapidly, are prepaid by
the client but pay the physician on a fee-for-service. The size
of the fee depends on the total utilization by physicians. Here
there is a balancing of forces for under- and over-utilization:
over-utilization decreases the fee for each service; under-
utilization decreases the total fee income. Both systems will see
marked growth in the near future.

One of the most fruitful areas of advance might lie in
pricing and entrepreneurship. If one seriously reduced
physicians' compensation for secondary and tertiary care
functions and increased prices for primary care functions
(Equation 2B), letting supply-demand function reach equilibrium, one might see rapid changes in care trends. More effort might go into Equation 2A functions, those of primary
care or office visits rather than into 2B functions such as oper-

ations and tests. Specialization might lose some of its appeal.

Entrepreneurship is appearing as large organizations are being developed to provide health care. These organizations will obviously begin to compete for enrollment, and will also compete for price. The artificial nature of hospital pricing will be open to challenge, particularly the capricious pricing of activities within the hospital to support various other functions; for example, overpricing in pharmacy, laboratory, and x-ray department to meet deficits in the operating room. The padding in one area to support "loss leaders" in another is not always equitable for patients, physicians, and third-party payers. As light is brought to this area, all three parties will complain and pricing may be opened up.

Prices and the medical-health care market have not escaped the scrutiny of the Wage and Price Boards.[39] After the initial freeze, decisions will continue to influence this market. On the wage side, added income will come through increased productivity. It will be interesting to see the Board deal with productivity in health care, a much more difficult struggle here than in industry in general, but one that may be vastly more rewarding for the citizen. In addition, the Wage Board has indicated that despite freezes in wages, there will be no limits in fringe benefits. This is not unlike the World War II situation that gave such an impetus to health insurance as a fringe benefit. The freedom to increase such benefits will shift further the burden of health care to industry and to the insurance company. The new infusion of capital into the health industry will be an incentive for large health care organizations and industrialists as well as insurance carriers to form partnerships. Each will be out for a hard bargain.

The demand-generating capacity of the physician is coming under direct scrutiny by peer groups, utilization committees, insurance companies, group practice organizations, medical foundations, industrialists, and insurance commissioners. The consumer guide for surgical care published by the Commissioner of Insurance of Pennsylvania is only one example.[40] The San Joaquin Valley Foundation review program is an excellent illustration of a physician-developed program to approach review of production functions in medical care.[41]

CONCLUSIONS

The medical-health care market, like all markets, is open to analysis with the techniques of modern economics. It is obvious that it is highly distorted, both because of the nature of the product and tradition. These distorting factors as they are reviewed by the physician and the client will become less powerful forces, and the market will be able to seek realistic balances that will favor the consumer and lessen his stress. One of the most fruitful areas for seeking a rational solution would be a critical attack on the problems of pricing.

NOTES

1. H. M. Somers, "Financing of Medical Care in the United States," *New England Journal of Medicine* 275 (1966):702-709.
2. W. L. Kissick, "Health Policy Directions for the 1970s," *NEJM* 282 (1970): 1343-1354.
3. D. P. Rice, B. S. Cooper, "National Health Expenditures 1929-71," *Social Security Bulletin* (January 1972), pp. 3-4.
4. B. Abel-Smith, "An International Study of Health Expenditure," *Public Health Paper 32* (Geneva: World Health Organization, 1967).
5. A. M. Burgess, T. Colton, and O. L. Peterson, "Categorical Programs for Heart Disease, Cancer and Stroke," *NEJM* 273 (1965):533-536.
6. Fein Rashi, "On Measuring Economic Benefit of Health Programs, Nuffield Provincial Hospitals Trust and Josiah Macy, Jr. Foundation," ed. Gordon McLachlan and Thomas McKeown, *Medical History and Medical Care* (London: Oxford University Press, 1971).
7. Dorothy Rice, "Estimating the Cost of Illness," *Health Economics* Series 6 (Washington: Government Printing Office, 1966).
8. Richard Gill, *Economics and the Private Interest* (Pacific Palisades, California: Goodyear Publishing Company, 1970), p. 4.
9. Victor Fuchs, "Health Care and the United States Economic System: An Essay in Abnormal Psychology," *Milbank Memorial Fund Quarterly* 40 (April 1972):211-237.
10. Victor Fuchs, p. 230.
11. H. L. Smith, "Two Lines of Authority Are One Too Many," *Modern Hospital* 84 (March 1955):59-64.
12. Kenneth Arrow, "Uncertainty and the Welfare Economics of Medical Care," *American Economic Review* 43 (December 1963):941-973.
13. E. A. Suchman, "Stages of Illness and Medical Care," *Journal of Health and Social Behavior* 6 (1965):114-118.
14. Arthur Owens, "The New Surge in Physicians Earning and Expenses," *Medical Economics* 46 (December 1969):83-88.
15. Richard Gill, p. 38.
16. M. J. Feldstein, "The Rising Prices of Physicians Services," *Review of Economics and Statistics* 52 (May 1970):121-133.
17. Interspecialty Committee of Massachusetts Medical Society: *1971 Massachusetts Relative Value Study.* Massachusetts Medical Society (Conversion Factors

came from telephone conversation with Dr. Gephart, Massachusetts Medical Society, October 1972).

18. R. L. Heilbroner, *Understanding Microeconomics* (Englewood Cliffs, N. J.: Prentice-Hall, Inc., 1968), pp. 1-2.

19. Committee on Cost of Medical Care: *Medical Care for the American People* (Chicago: University of Chicago Press, 1932), p. 9.

20. R. Andersen and D. W. Andersen, *A Decade of Health Services* (Chicago: University of Chicago Press, 1967), pp. 26-47.

21. National Center for Health Statistics: *Comment estimates from the Health Interview Survey*: United States, 1970. Vital and Health Statistics. PHS Pub. No. 1000-Series 10-No. 72. (Public Health Service, Washington, D.C., May 1972).

22. J. Hart, "Inverse Care Law," *Lancet* 1 (February 1971):405-412.

23. Committee on Cost of Medical Care, ed. Allan Peebles, *A Survey of Medical Facilities of Shelby County, Indiana*. (Washington, D.C. Committee on Cost of Care, 1929).

24. W. A. Reed and J. L. Ford, "Outpatient Clinic for Surgery," *Medical World News* 12 (1971):38.

25. H. C. Mather, N. C. Pearson, R. Lq. Read (D. B. Shaw, G. R. Steed, M. G. Thorne, S. Jones, C. J. Guerrier, C. D. Erant, P. M. McHugh, N. R. Chowdbury, M. H. Jafary, T. J. Wallace), "Acute Myocardial Infarction: Home and Hospital Treatment," *British Medical Journal* 3 (1971):334-338.

26. J. E. Harpur, W. T. Conner, M. Hamilton (R. J. Kellett, H. J. B. Galbraith, J. J. Murray, J. H. Swallow, G. A. Rose), "Controlled Trial of Early Mobilization and Discharge From Hospital in Uncomplicated Myocardial Infarction," *Lancet* 2 (1971): 1331-1334.

27. B. S. Bloom, O. L. Peterson, S. P. Martin, "Radiation Therapy in New Hampshire, Massachusetts, and Rhode Island: Output and Cost," *New England Journal of Medicine* 286 (1972): 189-194.

28. Richard Gill, p. 48.

29. Richard Gill, p. 48.

30. O. L. Peterson, A. M. Burgess, R. Berfenstram (B. Smedley, R. L. F. Logan, and R. J. C. Pearson), "What is Value for Money in Medical Care," *Lancet* 1 (1967): 771-776.

31. C. J. Hitch and R. M. McKean, *The Economics of Defense in the Nuclear Age* (New York: Atheneum 1967), pp. 105-133.

32. F. Smith, "Cost Effectiveness and Cost Benefit Analyses for Public Health Programs," *Public Health Reports* 83 (November 1968):899-906.

33. Alfred Yankauer, J. P. Connelly and J. J. Feldman, "Pediatric Practice in the United States," *Pediatrics* 45 (supp.) pp. 521-554.

34. Herbert E. Klarman, *The Economics of Health* (New York: Columbia University Press, 1965).

35. C. E. Lewis, B. A. Resnik, "Nurse Clinics and Progressive Ambulatory Patient Care," *New England Journal of Medicine* 227 (1967):1236-1241.

36. H. K. Silver, J. A. Hecker, "The Pediatric Nurse Practitioner and the Child Health Association: New Types of Health Professional," *Journal of Medical Education* 45 (1970):171-176.

37. Carnegie Commission on Higher Education: *Higher Education and the Nation's Health: Policy for Medical and Dental Education* (New York: McGraw Hill, 1970), pp. 55-59.

38. Alfred Yankauer, pp. 537-539.

39. *Economic Controls Report*, p. 9904 (Washington: Commerce Cleaning House, Inc., July 14, 1972).

40. H. S. Denenberg, *A Shopper's Guide to Surgery: Fourteen Rules on How to Avoid Unnecessary Surgery* (Harrisburg: The Pennsylvania Insurance Dept., 1972).

41. R. Saserly, C. E. Hopkins, "A Medical Society-Sponsored Comprehensive Medical Care Program," *Medical Care* 5 (1967):234-248.

AN EXPERIENCE WITH
INTERPROFESSIONAL EDUCATION

George Szasz

Interprofessional, Interdisciplinary and Health Team Education are terms currently used to denote modes of inter-relationships of the formal education of an increasing number of health care professionals, technologists and their associates and assistants. The experiences in this field at the University of British Columbia seem unique because extraordinary efforts have been made at that institution to inter-relate the administration of the various health professional schools and to create a common physical and educational milieu for the work of faculty members and students.

One segment of these efforts—the promotion of educational innovations—will be focused on here. The unfolding events are described from a historical perspective which includes, unavoidably, some personal views and biases. These might serve to indicate, however, that the work of the last few years has been filled with commitments, hopes, and aspirations; successes and setbacks.

THE BACKGROUND

Approximately one thousand students are enrolled and close to four hundred faculty members work in the faculties and schools or departments of medicine, nursing, dentistry, dental hygiene, pharmaceutical sciences, rehabilitation therapy (occupational and physiotherapy), social work, nutritional sciences and clinical psychology at the University of British Columbia.

These health professional faculties and schools are administered independently of each other and formulate their own educational policies. As can be expected, differences exist in the prerequisites for admission; the length of training; the extent and nature of the utilization of community and hospital resources for education; students' freedom or lack of it in the selection of courses; the time-tabling arrangements; the teaching load; the research interest; the facilities for postgraduate training; the methods of administration within the various schools; and the powers vested in the Deans and heads of schools.

In the early 1960s a complex of new buildings, dedicated primarily to training of medical students, was in the process of planning. Recognizing the emerging health manpower problems, Dean John F. McCreary suggested that the plans be expanded to provide a common physical milieu for the education of all the health professional students enrolled at the University of British Columbia.

It seemed to those of us who were involved in planning for this new facility that one of the major requirements for the future was to expand the influence of the diminishing number of primary care physicians. If this were indeed the case, it seemed important to plan in such a way that the facility could be used for training assistants to the physicians as well as for training physicians themselves. But who would become the assistants to the physician in the provision of primary health care? Could we rely on the already understaffed professions of nursing, rehabilitation therapy, social work, clinical psychology and the like to assist in this phase of the work as they have assisted in the hospital? Or would we need to train an entirely new type of individual, someone akin to the medical corpsman who has so successfully expanded the influence of the physician in military medicine? Because the design of the training facility need not differ greatly in any case, we elected to beg the question. We decided to attempt in the first instance to *integrate the teaching of the existing health professions* in such a way that they might better understand and appreciate what *each professional group could contribute*.[1]

The proposed attempt to purposefully interrelate the education of health professionals was first called "interdisciplinary education." However, many faculty members felt that this term implied an integration of basic science and clinical departments; so eventually "Interprofessional Education in the Health Sciences" was selected as a descriptive title.

Although the anticipation that future health care services will likely be provided by "teams" of collaborating health professionals was basic in the move toward Interprofessional Education, there was no agreement among the schools—and no agreement between faculty members of individual schools—on what the nature of these teams might be. Sidestepping this issue, the Committee of Deans and heads of schools established a Committee on Interprofessional Education in the Health Sciences for the purpose of finding ways and means of preparing students for "collaborative service relationships."

COMMITTEE ON INTERPROFESSIONAL EDUCATION

The Committee was composed of assistant and associate professor-level faculty members representing each of the health professional schools. It appeared reasonable for the Committee to try first to identify the barriers to collaboration and to understand the effects of these barriers on professional practice; then to generate ideas about ways and means of bringing these problems to the students' attention; to try out some of these methods in experimental programs, and finally, to submit the successful programs to the scrutiny of the Committee of Deans and, after approval, to assist the schools in the process of incorporation of new programs.

BARRIERS BETWEEN PROFESSIONS

The Committee has not been able to identify specific insurmountable obstacles between professions that would in themselves, with any certainty, lead to inadequate health care or that could not be overcome through adequate communication. It has found, however, some objective (and more subjective) evidence of differences between the various health professions that could impede adequate communication between members of the various health professions, contribute to misunderstanding and distrust, and maintain ignorance of each others' accomplishments and potentialities.

Some of these differences appear to be social or psychological in origin; others seem to be problems of economics and education. The Committee found that differences exist between the goals, training and technology of the various professions; in fact, these exist not only between professions but within professions as well. In medicine, the divergent orientations of surgery and psychiatry may serve as an example; within nursing, this difference in orientation is illustrated in the conflict between nursing education and nursing service; in rehabilitation, one may find a difference in orientation between physiotherapists and occupational therapists. Besides these differences, the status of some of the other professions in the health field is considerably below that of the physician, and even below that of certain occupations requiring comparable education and responsibility. The disparity in status is reflected in the differences in income and in the varying degrees of enthusiasm and motivation manifested in the work of some of the professionals.

In addition, certain social and psychological factors outside the professions place obstacles in the way of effective professional cooperation. The public tends to hold certain attitudes and beliefs regarding medicine, nursing, social work and the other health professions. The work of the physician tends to be regarded by many, including those in some of the health professions, as a glamorous activity in which the physician is leading a battle against disease.

In this context the Committee found that many professions have difficulty in projecting desirable up-to-date images to the public. The social worker's past image as an almoner has not yet been erased, the image of the pharmacist as a drug store propietor appears to be fixed, the image of the nurse as a competent modern professional person has still not been fully accepted, and the rehabilitation therapist is still often referred to as the kindly "rheumatic nurse." Because of these difficulties, the position of the various health professionals within the group that may cooperate is uncertain, and even the image of the physician either as a consultant or as a leader of the team is debated more on emotional than on factual grounds.

Apart from these social and psychological obstacles, a number of economic and organizational factors require consideration as well. Some authorities suggest that economic self-interest is a motivating factor behind the issue of who performs what health service and that the fee-for-service method of financing of present day medical practice does not permit utilization of the expertise offered by various professionals. Related to these economic problems are the administrative structures of hospitals and official and voluntary health agencies that may also block communication and collaboration between professions.

The Committee found that a basic problem inherent in traditional education also contributes to the establishment of barriers. Traditionally, education in western societies has stressed competitive, non-cooperative principles. To compete successfully and get ahead of others, as indicated by examination marks and other rewards, has been regarded as a social value by students, teachers and parents alike. The perspectives set in the general education of the student and fostered during his professional education are difficult to change—particularly because there are few, if any, role models in the professional schools or in practice offering examples of the principles of cooperation.

EDUCATIONAL DILEMMA

It became obvious to the Committee that administrative, economic, social and educational factors all have important influence on the relationship of one profession to another. The Committee debated whether professional schools are the right instruments to counter these factors. It concluded that appropriate educational programs would at least foster communication between professionals and would help the students of various professions to formulate a common, comprehensive outlook on human problems—which in turn might lead to collaboration in the management of these problems.

A Tentative Model

After considerable discussion, the Committee proposed a very tentative outline for an "interprofessional" curriculum. The outline suggests four levels. The first level provides the "professional foundation." During the three to four months assigned to this level, all entering students study a community's health problems, observe the work of various health professionals and focus their attention upon the methods and processes of interaction between the patient and the helper. The second level of the curriculum is the "foundation of medicine," "foundation of nursing" and the "foundation" of other professions. This level consists of a survey of the special knowledge and skills of each profession. Sharing the learning experiences between groups occurs if it is economically worthwhile, or otherwise justified. Courses within this level are oriented toward the unique needs of medical, nursing or other practices. Within medicine, for example, the students may start at the bedside studying the symptoms, signs and the physiological and biochemical changes brought about by stress; then study the various physical, social and psychological agents producing stress; then observe the pathological changes brought about by these, as seen in the laboratory and on the wards of hospitals and in the community. The time duration of this level necessarily varies with each faculty.

The detailed study of specific subjects contained in the second level is shifted to the third level: "health sciences in depth." At this level a large number of courses are offered by various schools. The subject matter may involve anatomy, behavioural sciences, the history of medical or health sciences, internal medicine, nursing practice, hospital administration and drug distribution systems. After consulting with advisers the students of the various schools select subjects for intensive study according to their interests, ability and needs. After the completion of three or four three-monthly periods in the third level, the student enters the last level: "health sciences in practice." In this level the students become responsibly involved in the team care of patients, and they also assume responsibilities for the teaching of lower-year students of the other professions. Throughout each of these levels the student also has responsibilities within community and treatment institutions and in various models of traditional and experimental systems of primary health care services.

This curriculum model was discussed with many department heads and faculty members. Although certain aspects of the outline were looked upon with interest, the model was rejected as the basis of a united educational policy for the health professional schools. The exercise, however, proved to be useful because it sparked a dialogue among the members of various faculties. Difficulties resulting from vagueness of educational objectives, lack of role models, inflexible timetables, conservatism, distrust between professions and failure to perceive emerging needs were discussed, and various approaches to the resolution of some of these problems were debated.

INTERPROFESSIONALIZATION

The Committee was not discouraged. Although it abandoned the proposed curriculum outline as the means of achieving collaborative relationships, it maintained that for any change to occur in health professional practice, students and practitioners alike will have to enlarge the scope of their current professional outlook. Specifically, the Committee felt that students graduating from any of the health professional schools or faculties of the University of British Columbia should demonstrate, through their behaviour, evidence of having become "interprofessionalized." The result of this process would mean an expansion of the behaviour now expected from a health professional to include: 1) increased awareness of the need for a comprehensive approach to a broad spectrum of human problems; 2) knowledge of the aids available from members of the other professions; 3) understanding of the attitudes, values and methods of those providing these aids; and, 4) the ability to appropriately utilize aid from other professions in whatever organizational relation health care services may be offered.

As the Committee contemplated these tentative educational objectives, it found itself at a fork in the road. Was it the Committee's role to define what "increased awareness" means, list the aids that are available, describe the attitudes and values that might be possessed by various groups of people, and outline at what depth principles of group dynamics should be practised? Or should the Committee cause involvement of students and staff alike in a variety of educational experiences so that they might consider and clarify the objectives and devise methods whereby these might be reached?

OFFICE OF INTERPROFESSIONAL EDUCATION

The latter procedure was chosen because the Committee felt that a critical mass of the faculty must eventually be in favour of major program innovations. Accordingly, the Committee recommended to the Deans that an Office of Inter-professional Education be established for the purposes of stimulating the interest and involvement of both faculty members and students in programs likely to lead to "interpro-fessionalization." The Committee would remain in an advis-ory role to the Office and the Chairman became the Director of the Office. These terms were accepted and an Office of Interprofessional Education in the Health Sciences was estab-lished in 1968.

At the time the Office was established, it appeared prudent to place it outside of the jurisdiction of all schools and to make it into an administratively powerless, politically non-threat-ening, academically non-competitive agency. Financing was obtained from sources largely outside of university funds.

These cautious arrangements were necessary for two reasons. First, at the time of the establishment of the Office, the administrative relationship between the various schools and the building program were still in the elementary stages of their development. As the Health Sciences Centre adminis-tration emerged, a coalition type of relationship was estab-lished among the heads of the health professional schools. A Coordinating Committee was formed, and a Coordinator

—appointed by the President of the University—became the chairman of the Committee. The Coordinator has no budgetary or academic authority over any of the schools. The budget of his office is independent from the budgets of the health professional schools, and it is derived from both university and grant sources. In this rather unique administrative arrangement, the Coordinator is neither an executive officer of the President of the University nor the representative of any of the heads of the schools to the President.

The Coordinator works with the Coordinating Committee on the short- and long-range planning of shared building facilities, and he is responsible to the Committee for the management of the shared educational, research and service activities of the Health Professional Schools, including the administration of the integrated aspects of continuing education programs for the health professions. The Coordinator also works with the Deans and heads of schools to have the Health Sciences Centre identified as a functional unit within the university and to establish a province-wide voice for health professional education.

The arrangements prepared for the Office of Interprofessional Education therefore had to parallel the development of the Coordinator's Office. As the logical follow-up, the Office has recently become a Division of the Coordinator's Office, joining other divisions which serve the Coordinator in various advisory capacities.

The second reason for placing the Office of Interprofessional Education outside the jurisdiction of the schools was that a number of faculty members expressed their concern over the interrelation of educational programs. Some felt that this meant a dilution of existing teaching programs, others suggested that the "interprofessional" goals were not any different from what the various schools were aiming for already. A few faculty members looked upon the activities of the Committee on Interprofessional Education as a form of unwelcome interference in the schools' internal operation. In addition, a number of faculty members questioned the authority of the Coordinating Committee in the area of curriculum developments. These, they argued, were the domain

of the individual schools. In light of these factors, the shelter-   ·
ing of the Office had become a necessity.

Initial Activities

The activities of the Office—and later Division—reflect a
series of reactions to the difficulties inherent in a process of
"gentle persuasion" of faculty members caught up in debates
over administrative organizations, planning of physical
facilities, and making changes in their own curricula. The
latter activities have been—and are—the most difficult ones to
accommodate. Clearly, faculty members have perceived the
need for change in the educational programs of their schools;
but their perception of the needs and their approach to the
resolution have been along the lines of uniprofessional rather
than interprofessional activities.

The first objective of the Director was to identify faculty
members and students who might be sympathetic to the principles of interprofessionalization. The second objective was to
work with these faculty members and students on various
experimental programs to discover what the content and
methodology of these might be and how they might fit into the
existing curricula. The third objective was to establish a
number of service functions which might make the Office
—and later the Division—a desirable part of the administrative structure of all the schools.

Faculty Involvement

For these purposes, and without prior formulation of any
long-range plans, the Office initiated a series of brief educational programs which either illustrated examples of cooperation among health care professionals or pointed to the need
for closer collaboration. As one example of cooperation
among professionals, a program on mental retardation was
initiated, and the joint contribution of geneticists,
psychologists, physicians, nurses, rehabilitation therapists,
pharmacologists, teachers and others to the patients and their
families was demonstrated. In another program a mother

related the anguish and suffering which arose following the birth of her mongoloid child. In this case, the lack of collaboration between the medical and nursing staff and the exclusion of other professionals who could have contributed to the welfare of the child and the family could be clearly identified as causes of the family's suffering.

These and similar programs were planned, conducted and evaluated by faculty members and students, all serving in a voluntary capacity. The programs took place outside of the regular curricula. The Office looked after the physical arrangements and subsidized the relatively minor expenditures; it only insisted that in all the programs the comprehensive nature of human problems were to be emphasized and the contribution—or lack of them—of the various health professions to the assessment and treatment or rehabilitation of the individual, the family or the community were to be demonstrated.

The programs touched a responsive chord in the students, and as the number of students attending these initial programs increased, an atmosphere of enthusiasm developed among them for interrelated educational experiences. At the same time it became apparent that many faculty members were also interested in making a contribution to these programs. It was obvious that many faculty members were concerned with the lack of collaboration between professions, but because of their confining time-table arrangements, the often narrow departmental teaching objectives, and plain overwork, they were unable to share with the students the knowledge and experience derived from their own collaborative relationships with other professionals.

Faculty members from rehabilitation, social work and nursing appeared to be the most interested in the programs; those medical faculty members who attended the various events usually had an interest in some aspect of community medicine. The faculty members who participated in planning some of the programs seemed to have a strong motivation to present their professions in a good light. Many of these faculty members had degrees in more than one field (for example, nursing and education) and had arrived at this university relatively recently. Some of the participating faculty members expressed hostility toward members of the medical profession, but interestingly, not against medical faculty members. Participating faculty members did not form any organization to promote the interprofessional cause; in fact, when challenged by their colleagues on the practicality of various forms of collaboration, a number of previously interested faculty members dropped out of the activities.

LATER DEVELOPMENTS

The Office of Interprofessional Education continued to offer conferences, student group projects, patient management exercises, lecture programs, field trips and the like. All these programs emphasized that health professionals cannot afford to neglect the formulations of other professionals in the management of their patients and clients. In the meantime, a few shared programs were accepted into the regular curricula of some of the schools. Some of these were also initiated by faculty members through their departmental and school structures independently.

An interesting example of the tenuous and delicate nature of interrelated programs is the participation of the School of Nursing in a first-year medical course over a 5-year period. This course, entitled "Preclinical Sessions," was basically an introduction to human growth and development, as well as to interviewing, and included discussions of problems relating to the various age groups in the context of the family setting. Each student was assigned to a family with young children to permit observation of the growth and development of children and the interpersonal relations of a growing family. The course consisted of 30 lecture hours and about 45 hours of seminar-type small group meetings in addition to the meetings with the families.

The Director of the Office suggested to the school of nursing that participation in this course might be of some value both to nursing and medical students. The school of nursing assigned 5 volunteer students from the penultimate year of their course. The students made quite a contribution to the course, and faculty members of the school of nursing observing them felt that the course was of considerable value to their students—particularly in bringing them into close working relationship with medical students. The school of nursing sent 6 volunteer students the following year, and several faculty members from the school were invited to participate in the seminar discussion. In the following year, the school of nursing included this course as a formal requirement for students in their penultimate year. Faculty members became co-tutors and shared responsibilities for seminars with their medical counterparts. The nursing and medical tutors formed a curriculum committee and made recommendations for the next year.

In the next year the course became an elective subject for any year in the school of nursing. Although the tutors were pleased with certain aspects of the course, they felt that the nursing students were more advanced in their understanding of families than the medical students. They hoped that a number of lower year students might elect this course, but because of time-table problems, this was not possible.

At this point the school of nursing withdrew from the course. In the meantime, however, the course director and the involved medical faculty members came to appreciate the contribution made by the nursing faculty members, and they started to reach out for public health nurses, rehabilitation therapists and social workers from the community to act as co-tutors. At the present, students and faculty observers from rehabilitation medicine and pharmaceutical sciences are testing the applicability of this program to their curriculum and estimating the demands on the staff if involvement is found to be desirable.

In contrast to the active part played by the Office of Interprofessional Education in the "Preclinical Sessions," the Office had little to do with negotiations going on between, for example, the medical and dental faculties with regard to their joint basic medical science program. Similarly, the department of psychiatry conducted its own negotiations with the school of rehabilitation medicine when a common program was being prepared for medical and rehabilitation medicine

students, and the faculty of pharmaceutical sciences and the
school of nursing preferred to make their own arrangements
with some of the basic science departments. In most of these
instances, however, the educational activities were not "jointly
planned, developed, carried out and evaluated by faculty
members of the involved schools," rather the courses offered
by one school were made "available" to students of other
schools.

STUDENT INVOLVEMENT

Considerable energy was expended to involve students in
interprofessional activities. The first programs occurred in
that time period which was marked by student unrest on
various campuses. Although the University of British Columbia was relatively quiet during those turbulent years of the late
1960s, a large number of students were excited and eager to
participate in programs which appeared humanistic in their
orientation and often involved some form of community service as well. A group of students formed an interprofessional
organization, and generated their own programs. Interestingly, this group first felt that the interprofessional activities
promoted by the Office were unrealistic because they were
more or less limited to health professionals. The students
expanded their organization, and included, among others,
students from the school of theology and the faculty of education.

In each of the last four years the Office—and later the
Division—maintained a slightly different form of relationship
with this student group. In the first year, strong leadership
was offered to students, including frequent meetings, social
activities and travel opportunities for students. In the second
year, a recent graduate of the school of nursing was employed
as an "assistant" in charge of promotion of specific student
projects. In the third year, two faculty members for the school
of social work were engaged on a part-time basis to assist in the
management of such projects as camps for emotionally dis-
turbed and crippled children. Their expertise in management of group processes was also utilized. In the fourth year,

only a distant support was offered to the students. Secretarial services, financing of projects and so forth were easily available, but the personal leadership and assistance of the previous years was less evident.

Experiences at the University of British Columbia seem to indicate that strong leadership combined with the day-to-day services offered by an "assistant" is needed to bring about active student participation in innovative activities.

However, in the last year or so it has appeared wiser to tone down the student activities. One reason for this was that some students became so involved in the projects that their academic progress began to suffer. A few active, innovative students actually dropped out of school. It is of course difficult to explain what happened in these instances, but frustration with the present system of education may have been a causal factor. The Director felt that, however indirectly and inadvertently, those students were being used to foster change in their faculty. The second reason was that students started to question the validity of some of the interprofessional ideas when they did not see their own professors applying them in patient care settings. Interestingly, these doubts started to appear as the student mood settled on the campuses.

Today, the student organization functions independently from the Division of Interprofessional Education. There is frequent informal contact between the students and the office, and students are able to receive rapid support (finances, secretarial help, stationery, meeting rooms, etc.) if they generate ideas for programs which are within the desired objectives of the Division of Interprofessional Education. Representatives of the student organization sit on committees responsible for the management of common facilities, such as the Instructional Resources Centre which houses the majority of classrooms and common rooms.

SERVICE FUNCTIONS

Gradually, four areas emerged as territories for the activities of the Division of Interprofessional Education.

Interprofessional Education Affairs. In the area of interprofessional affairs, the Division assisted or stimulated the development of over 40 programs of short or long duration. In the course of these it tried out the relative effectiveness of various forms of "mixing" of students, offered financial or technical support to programs that had "interprofessionalization" potentials, assisted with audio-visual facility utilization and planning of shared facilities and space allocation, and offered assistance with "newsletter" information services to students as well as a bibliography service on interprofessional relationships.

The Division plays an indirect role in the programs of the Family Practice Unit and the Community Health Centre—two of the Health Sciences Centre demonstration units. While all policies and plans are developed by the staff of these units and negotiations for utilization are conducted by heads of schools, the Office assists the staff of these units through consultations. The units are also the scene of several interprofessional activities. The Division has also coordinated and managed several courses for various faculties. These courses were not necessarily interprofessional but were given by a large number of instructors from various departments. The central service for time-table allocation, notification of the instructors, and collating notes, has proved to be useful.

Student Interprofessional Affairs. In the area of student interprofessional affairs, the Division assists students with technical support of their developing interprofessional organization and with support of such student programs as the development of national/international connections, newsletter services and health care oriented summer job opportunities. The Division was instrumental in establishing a summer camp for disabled children, operated in its entirety by health professional students. In addition, the Division has participated in vocational guidance programs for undergraduates seeking a health professional career.

Research. A third area emerged as the need for research about the nature of interprofessional education became obvious. Formulation of interprofessional objectives, testing of teaching methods for their relative effectiveness and development of evaluation instruments are examples of some of the probings. A need was identified for new types of architectural arrangements of service areas to be used by teams of students in the course of their clinical training.

An attempt was made to develop a new type of exam to test the *outcome* of the shared work of the students. For example, in a program where medical and nursing students operated—under supervision—a teenage sexual advice and birth control clinic, attempts were made to evaluate the joint performance of the students by observing patients' behaviour after the visit. The difficulties were too great, however, so a paper and pencil problem-solving exam was devised. In this type of exam the focus is not only on the students' medical or nursing knowledge, but also on their understanding of each others' capabilities and of the need for considering each others' formulations about the patient and his environment. One of these exams developed for medical students starts like this:

Parents rush into an emergency room of a 200-bed hospital. Intern is not available. Child is in parent's arms, looks about 5 years of age; gasping for breath.

Nurse would now: (choose only one of the following)
  1. take brief history
  2. call family doctor
  3. examine child
  4. sedate child
  5. call supervisor

Few of the medical students mark 1 as the correct answer, for they do not perceive a nurse's enquiry as "taking brief history." As the exam questions and answers unfold, the nurse's abilities are brought into focus, and if the medical students insist on excluding the nurse from the assessment and management tasks, the pathways of the programmed exam may bring him to a point where the child dies because of the unnecessary delays in management created by ignoring of the signals of another health professional.

A similar exam has been developed for the nursing student, using the same story but emphasizing the need for her to take action based on her knowledge and skills. These tests offer promise both as teaching tools and as an evaluation instrument, but they are still in the early phase of their development.

Apart from such exams, new insights are also needed into student attitudes, the manner of the development of their professional image, and the impact of interprofessional education on these; causes of attrition, and, of course, long-range evaluation of the behaviour of students educated in an interprofessional milieu.

Liaison Activities. Liaison activities including links with various health care agencies, particularly with continuing education organizations, emerged as the fourth area for legitimate activities of the Division of Interprofessional Education. A "public relations" type of activity, including addresses to student groups, professional and business organizations, voluntary and official agencies, is also being maintained.

EVALUATION

Some attempt has been made to evaluate each program offered under the auspices of the Committee on Interprofessional Education. The methods of evaluation vary, but usually include paper and pencil tests, exams, attendance records, and such vague indices as the length of applause during or following presentations, comments by faculty members, requests for return presentations, news of the program filtering to students of other classes in the schools and others. Official acceptance of certain presentations as part of the curriculum is also considered as a form of evaluation by faculty members as are the occasions when students do not appear at or in fact walk out on a program.

In general, several of these "instruments" are used together to find out whether the student's awareness of the need for a comprehensive approach to certain human problems has increased, whether he has gained new understanding or insights about the contributions which other professionals might make to the assessment and management of these problems, and whether the student's ability to work in group situations has increased as the consequence of his participation in a particular program or set of programs.

Evaluation of the programs has proved to be exceedingly difficult. No attempt was made to estimate any behavioural changes in terms of the long-range objectives. The experiences gathered over the last few years have served, however, to suggest some general conclusions about the "fit" of the content and the methodology of interprofessional programs into the regular curricula of the various schools.

THE FIT OF THE CONTENT

It appears now that the content presented in the framework of interprofessional programs does not always fit in well with the curriculum. One reason for this is that the presentations tend to arouse anxieties in faculty members and sometimes also in the students. The presentations often suggest in no uncertain terms that there are weaknesses in the health care delivery system and that these are sometimes caused by professional isolation and disregard for the formulations of others.

A second reason for the ill fit is that the content of the programs is derived from several disciplines. This contrasts with most curricula for they are usually based on a sequential or parallel, but not on an integrated presentation of subjects. A third reason for the ill fit is sometimes traceable to the students' preconceived notions of what they should learn. Of course, students often pick up these notions in their respective schools (sometimes from the type of exam), but many enter the professional school with perspectives which make it difficult for them to accept interprofessional content as "relevant."

In general, students of the first two years of medicine show more interest in interprofessional programs than students of the last two years. Interestingly, the reverse is true of students of nursing, pharmacy and dentistry. In contrast, students of rehabilitation medicine are keenly interested throughout their education, and students of social work show little if any interest.

It appears that medical students in their early years really desire the clinical orientation provided by interprofessional programs. As a price, they also accept the presence of others in these programs. Later they identify themselves with clinicians, and consider interprofessional programs a "dilution" of their education.

Nursing, pharmacy and dental students become aware of their own potential in patient care procedures toward the end of their training and only then become keenly interested in interprofessional activities. Rehabilitation students are taught the importance of team approach from the first day of their classes. Not seeing this approach being practised outside of rehabilitation institutions, they are eager to foster interprofessional activities. The interest of social work students seems to be limited because they tend to perceive interprofessional activities proceeding along a "medical model" and feel that this model (physician the "captain") is not appropriate any longer.

THE FIT OF THE METHODS

Mixing was thought to be the principal methodology of interprofessional educational programs. It appears now that, in general, students and faculty react positively to students of another profession in their classes only if they receive an explanation of the need to have common learning experiences.

Mixing might be desirable if it offers: 1) a visible proof that faculty members and students of many professions need to share certain areas of knowledge and skills; 2) an opportunity for faculty members to work together on the planning and evaluation of various programs; and 3) an economical method of presentation.

Mixing can become undesirable if: 1) the planning and evaluation of the program is not shared by faculty members; and 2) students are not prepared for such interrelationships.

In these instances students at best ignore each other; at worst they resent the presence of the others. It appears that students are afraid that their learning experiences are being "diluted."

Mixing of students is relatively well accepted in the be-, havioural and social sciences, public health and, to a certain extent, psychiatric content areas—much less so in the basic biomedical science areas, and least in the clinical areas. In general, problems related to mixing seem to be a reflection of traditional territorial imperatives of various professions. The student's interest and performance in a mixed program seem to be directly proportional to his chosen profession's traditional interest (or lack of it) in the content area of the programs.

Associated with the principle of mixing, the Committee believed that sharing physical facilities, both in the classroom and coffee room areas and in clinical facilities, is a necessary vehicle of interprofessional education, shared facilities being "identifiable service units consisting of physical space, equipment and service personnel, which are fully or partially utilized for interprofessional activities and which are administered by the Coordinating Committee of the Health Sciences Centre." There is no evidence at hand yet to indicate the value of physical space sharing in the pursuit of interprofessional objectives. There is, however, good evidence that the process of joint planning for and maintenance procedures of such facilities provides for a forum of interprofessional exchange.

JOINT PROGRAM PLANNING

The Office has insisted that interprofessional programs are "those which are planned, carried out and evaluated by faculty members of two or more schools for students of two or more schools." This principle is respected by faculty members, but does not fit in well with the existing administration of the schools. A department or a school must be responsible for each course. Policy formulations, budgeting and staff allocation are the prerogatives of departments and schools. Consequently, even if well-meaning faculty members are able to cooperate, departmental or school pressures may negate all their work. Because of the lack of clearcut arrangements between schools, many willing faculty members have to add extra time to their usually already overloaded time-table if they wish to participate in interprofessional ventures.

EXAMS

Interprofessional exams, both in the form of paper and pencil tests and as observation of clinical performance of teams, are feasible, although as yet very awkward. The major value of these exams is that they make the students think not only about the knowledge but also about the manner of behaviour expected of them. It is precisely because it is still not entirely clear just exactly what is efficient and effective that these attempts at evaluation are so difficult. It is quite likely that the recently developed "problem-oriented records" may prove to be valuable teaching tools for interprofessional education.

AUDIO-VISUAL SUPPORT

When attempts are being made to establish common attitudes to certain problem areas, emotion-producing movies or television tapes or even sound recordings depicting human conditions seem to be a valuable approach to generating similar emotions in a mixed class of students. The students tend to feel "we are all in this together" or "how can we all help?" Brief segments of video-taped scenes depicting activities of patients suffering from such disorders as emphysema, chronic heart failure or arthritis appear to bring relevance to students who do not usually have contact with patients but who study certain aspects of pathology or medicine.

VOLUNTARY PROGRAMS

Electives or voluntary after hours and summertime programs have considerable value in bringing community health problems into focus for the students, provided that the students have some freedom to exercise their creativity and that guidance is available to them on a colleague (rather than student-faculty) basis. Volunteer activities appeared to be a greater success at the beginning of the interprofessional activities. In the last two years, however, there has been some lessening of student enthusiasm about various projects. The reason for this is hard to explain. In the last year, there has been definitely less personal leadership offered to students as part of the plan to discover the most desirable type of relationship between the Office and the student organization. However, in the last year or so there have also occurred a number of social changes which have perhaps channeled student interest to other endeavours.

DEMONSTRATION MODELS,
TEACHER ACTIVITIES AND BEHAVIOUR

One purpose of the Family Practice Unit, the Community Health Centre and similar demonstration projects is to offer an opportunity for the student to imitate collaborative forms of behaviour. There is, however, a problem with demonstration models, for they are often something unusual and not quite accepted by faculty members. As such, they often become targets of criticism which is frequently based on hearsay or fragmentary evidence.

The result is that students who enjoy working in the demonstration models may feel that they have to defend the model's personnel or the nature of the activities taking place there. This might not be an undesirable exercise except that most health care demonstration models have great difficulty in showing whether their method of operation is more effective, more efficient, professionally more satisfying or scientifically more justifiable than the methods practised by the large majority of the teaching staff. Under these circumstances, the students may become anxious and might find it easier to ignore the model and follow the examples set by the mainstream of faculty.

However, the demonstration by example of collaborative service relationships seems to be a most significant method of teaching the ways of working together. One could expect this, of course, for becoming and acting like a professional is, to a great extent, a matter of imitating the behaviour of one's teachers. The desirable teacher seems to be the one who through his behaviour gives clear evidence that professional behaviour is both alterable and perfectable.

The significant values that need to be conveyed to the students seem to be those of simple courtesy and of intellectual and social concern which go beyond the particular jurisdictional claim of the teacher's own profession. Some faculty members, however, seem to believe that revelation of such feelings is not appropriate in the context of academic environment.

Conclusions and Comments

In the course of the various activities, it became apparent that the principles to be woven through the interprofessional educational process are that professional behaviour is a significant variant in the delivery of effective and efficient health care services, and that the application of the scientific method to the selection of the appropriate behaviour pattern is a vital part of being a professional. The desired ways of collaboration among health professionals need to be demonstrated by faculty members who work on hospital wards, ambulatory care areas, in the home of patients or in community agencies. Students need to practice collaboration in the course of their clinical studies and internships.

To enable students to work and study together in various patient care areas, they all must possess some knowledge and certain skills in the various aspects of biological, medical and social sciences; in the techniques of interviewing and record keeping; and in the managerial aspects of health care. The necessary depth and extent of knowledge and skills is still unclear; it is, however, the minimum rather than the maximum level that needs to be determined. Whether the basic educational programs are conducted in one or several buildings and whether the students are mixed or not in their various courses seem to be of secondary importance.

The practical implications of these findings are that:
1) Increasing numbers of demonstration areas need to be

created. These units should be so organized that the work of each of the various professionals in the assessment, treatment, and rehabilitation and prevention of individual or community health care problems can be perceived. Architectural changes may be necessary in these units to accommodate more students.

2) There is an urgent need for increasing numbers of faculty members—particularly from other than the medical schools—to assume combined clinical-academic responsibilities, so that students may have contacts with an increasing number of role models.

3) Few if any new courses need to be introduced, but some established courses need to be made available to a number of faculties—perhaps at varying levels of depth.

4) The students' time-tables need to be freed somewhat in order to give them opportunities to participate in joint learning experiences outside of the formal curriculum.

5) A system of examination needs to be developed so that student teams instead of individuals may be evaluated on their competency in utilizing each others' knowledge in their care of patients.

6) Faculty members need assistance to develop trust in each other through gradual involvement in interprofessionally oriented academic and clinical activities. This attitude may be fostered if: a) department and school heads strongly endorse participation of faculty members and students in interprofessional programs; b) programs continue to be created and promoted by an agency—so that sympathetic faculty members can join in with ease; and c) contractual arrangements can be made with faculty members (and departments) for the preparation, conduct and evaluation of specified educational programs.

It is important to recognize that the development of objectives, content and methodology of the programs was influenced by features unique to the functioning of the various health professional schools at this university, the administrative structure of the Health Sciences Centre organization, and the personalities involved in the Committee and later Office and Division of Interprofessional Education. In general, confrontations were carefully avoided, and pleas were made for collaboration on intellectual and humanitarian grounds. Partly as a consequence, the programs, as they evolved, became relegated to the periphery, rather than the mainstream of the formal curricula of the various schools. A number of faculty members became enthusiastic about the developments and have become actively involved in a number of programs. Most have remained noncommital or viewed the activities with disdain.

The precise reasons for these attitudes are not clear. Perhaps the ideas inherent in interprofessional education are not timely yet; perhaps the assumption that "students who learn together will work together" is too idealistic; perhaps the educational priorities of the various schools lie elsewhere. In any case, in the last year it appeared necessary to decelerate the program development and to let other interprofessional issues come to the foreground. Debates about the nature and location of further patient care facilities, development of a problem-oriented, computerizable information system for the various health care institutions, and re-discussions of the overall goals of the Health Sciences Centre serve right now as the principal points of contact between the schools. It is expected that out of these debates and discussions will emerge agreements which will open the way for further interrelationship of the education of health professionals.

In the course of all these events, the sights have not been lowered. Those who are committed to the Health Sciences Centre educational principle believe that eventually the graduates of this centre will enter into types of working relationship with other professionals which will be based on an appreciation and understanding of the need for the utilization of each others' formulations in health care services.

NOTE

1. John F. McCreary, "The Health Team Approach to Medical Education," *Journal of the American Medical Association* 206, No. 7 (11 November 1968): 1554-1557.

THE DILEMMA IN
DENTAL EDUCATION

John W. Hein

Programs for the education of dental auxiliaries present an increasingly attractive opportunity for a wide variety of institutions of higher education to demonstrate the sincerity of their interest in relating to society's needs. This is good. If, however, these opportunities are to be realized in a way which will yield the greatest long-term usefulness, they must be grasped by those having an appreciation for the liabilities as well as the assets of the present situation. If this does not happen, there will be a great waste of human and material resources and, even more important, progress toward improved oral health for the American people will be hindered.

A comprehensive review of dental auxiliary education and utilization, published in the *Journal of the American Dental Association* in 1972, supports the conviction that this is no time to gloss over the challenges facing us on all sides.[1]

NATURE OF ORAL DISEASE

To understand the focus and motivations which are molding the future of dental auxiliary education one must first know something of the nature of oral disease, because in the final analysis the oral health problems of the nation will determine the nature of the dental profession and its dental manpower. If this simple truth seems to have escaped attention on occasion, it is only because the sheer magnitude of the oral health problem is so overwhelming.

Dentistry is in a very real sense dealing with a plague. In an excellent summary of the situation, Greene points out that the unmet dental needs in the country add up to the biggest and costliest problem in the whole field of health.[2] He shows that for all practical purposes few can hope to escape. Ninety-five percent of all Americans are attacked by dental caries. Sixty percent of young adults, 80 percent of the middle aged and 90 percent of those over 65 suffer from periodontal disease. Sixty percent of American children require orthodontic treatment, and for one out of five of these the condition is so serious as to be deforming or crippling. Hence, if one were to view the population of the United States from a satellite, it would be seen that oral disease blankets the land like a coat of paint. It is everywhere; the cabin in the Maine woods, the penthouse on Park Avenue, the farm house in Kansas, the sharecropper's cottage in Alabama or the beach house in Malibu all harbor a fair share of its victims. Since oral diseases are chronic and do not cure themselves, treatment and preventive care are needed everywhere by everyone.

Unfortunately, what is needed and what takes place are not the same thing. Most oral disease is left untreated and allowed to accumulate. Thus, as Greene points out, while we spend $4 billion a year on care, a $54-billion backlog of disease goes untreated. The tip of this iceberg of neglect is revealed by the current experience of the armed forces which must fill 850 tooth surfaces, extract 101 teeth and provide 59 bridges and dentures for every 100 able-bodied (sic) men accepted.

There is, of course, nothing new about this deplorable situation. Our country suffered from a national toothache from the moment it was colonized, and acceptance of the pain and discomfort of oral disease as just one more of life's inescapable burdens became a firmly entrenched national ethic. In large measure it has remained so to this day, even though several decades have been added to life expectancy, thus prolonging the misery and compounding the problem. Any doubts concerning the persistence of this ethic can be dispelled by a reading of recent government justifications for excluding dental care as a health benefit from any national health program. What was good enough for our forefathers is apparently still good enough for us.

It is true, of course, that antibiotics have largely eliminated the life-threatening aspects of dental neglect. Hence, if one wishes to discount the pain, discomfort, poor health and gradual loss of pleasant appearance which result from such neglect, it can be done without too much fear of courting a death-defying situation. Furthermore, one has some very definite dollars and cents benchmarks against which to make such personal discounts because dental care readily lends itself to pricing. Regretably, the cost of good dental health usually appears high in this equation because in most all instances the cost must also include the price of repairing years of accumulated neglect. But in all honesty, cost is only part of the answer. The other part is simply that most dental care requires professionally trained personnel to spend a great deal of time in personal contact with the patient. In short, the largest part of dental care, whether it is being provided by a dentist or a dental hygienist, involves surgical types of procedures.

The nature of oral disease clearly points to prevention as the ultimate solution of the problem. Unfortunately, the same factors which have contributed to a national willingness to live with the problem have hamstrung the search for effective preventive measures. For example, never during the past century has the annual support of dental research equaled one percent of the funds expended during the year for dental care. Indeed, until ten years ago the main research burden for solving the major oral health problems of the nation was carried by manufacturers of dentifrices and chewing gums.

While this situation would be incomprehensible in relation to any other disfiguring disease of pandemic proportions, it must be recognized as a unique aspect of the oral disease picture. It also follows that while one may hope that modest research efforts will lead to dramatic scientific breakthroughs in the near future, the wisest course will be to make plans based on current knowledge.

In summary, the paradoxical nature of the oral health problems of the nation can be encapsulated in one sentence: oral disease presents the biggest and costliest problem in the field of health, but don't take it too seriously!

For well over a century, dentistry and its manpower, educational programs, professional organizations and care delivery systems have been evolving under the shadow of this strange paradox. And, as might well be expected, much of the evolution has necessarily been in response to the lesser stimuli which arise from the demand for dental care rather than the larger stimulus which would have derived from considerations of need.

Progress in delivery of dental care has been remarkably meritorious under the circumstances, but some defects and peculiarities exist. They have great relevance for anyone wishing to understand the problems facing dental auxiliary education.

THE NATURE OF DENTISTRY

Because oral disease has always been a major health problem affecting the entire population, it has made good sense for dental education to be tailored to the production of competent practitioners in the shortest possible time. The decision to follow this mission-oriented path, which created a fundamental difference between dental and medical education, took place well over a hundred years ago and has been until recently one of the basic goals of dental education.

For the past fifty years the required course for practitioners has been four academic years in dental school after at least two years of predental work in college. This format has held true in spite of a steady increase in the knowledge and skills required to be a highly qualified general practitioner. One consequence of this pressure has been a gradual loss of self-confidence among many senior students which has resulted in an ever larger number electing to go on to some form of postdoctoral training before entering practice. A number of dental educators have encouraged this trend by deliberately lessening the intensity of clinical training given in the dental school and encouraging postdoctoral study.

The result of these factors is an ambivalent profession. The older generations of dentists are preoccupied with general dental care, while many among the newer generations view it as less important in relation to their own career goals. Both of these attitudes have great significance for those concerned with dental auxiliary education. Many holding the former more conservative attitude look on expanded roles for dental auxiliaries as a threat, while many of those holding the latter attitude welcome this development as a godsend. The present leaders of the profession are, of course, mainly from the older generation and they determine the present climate, but dental auxiliary education must begin preparing for a drastic change in the weather.

Because oral diseases are pandemic, it made good sense for the graduates of dental schools to filter out across the country-side and establish small offices situated close to target populations. At least, it made good sense as long as dental schools turned out self-confident, general-practice-oriented graduates; the population was not predominantly located in urban areas; and demand for care rather than need was the guiding factor.

The dental care delivery system which developed on this basis has been derisively called a "cottage industry," yet in many respects it fits the nature of oral disease far better than any other available system. It does, of course, have limitations. It will only permeate as far as demand (that is, *money*) will support it. Moreover, small dental practices are very sensitive to overhead costs and this limits their ability to adopt measures which will lead to greater productivity and lower costs. The use of dental auxiliaries is one of the most important of these measures; the inability of the present dental care delivery system to utilize them most effectively is not only one of the major problems facing the dental profession but the greatest obstacle in the path of dental auxiliary education.

Until very recently the production of dental auxiliary manpower was a modest effort geared to the modest demands generated by the small dental office type of care delivery system. The economics of the situation not only discouraged greater production of auxiliaries but actually discouraged efforts to develop formal or more meaningful programs. Minimally trained auxiliaries working for minimal wages was a satisfactory order of the day for a "cottage industry."

During the past decade the number of dental auxiliary programs for both dental hygienists and dental assistants has expanded explosively. The principal stimulus has been federal funding which encouraged the inclusion of dental auxiliary training programs in the burgeoning community college system. It should be understood, however, that this development was not entirely appreciated, encouraged or welcomed by the majority of the dental profession; many were not only quite happy with on-the-job training for dental assistants but were hoping that dental hygiene training might somehow be returned to a one-year program.

Thus, what became a powerful force for the formalization and advancement of dental auxiliary education has also become the seed for a serious future crisis. For clearly, unless the dental profession becomes much more ready, willing and able to absorb effectively the rapidly increasing numbers of highly motivated, highly skilled dental auxiliaries, the field of dental auxiliary education faces a depression. Heads of educational institutions, who have been encouraged by local dental groups to initiate dental auxiliary programs, may tend to dismiss this danger, but they should carefully reexamine the motives for the request. Was it based on a clearly expressed need for college trained dental auxiliaries and solid evidence that the graduates could be appropriately absorbed into the work force? Or did the request stem from such unexpressed reasons as an unwillingness to offer sufficient inducements to attract dental auxiliaries to the area or a hope that local overproduction would depress the wages of dental auxiliaries?

These are unkind questions, but they are not stated in unkindness to the dental profession. They are, instead, a frank expression of the unfavorable results to be expected when government-supported manpower programs become out of phase with the evolution of the field they are intended to serve.

A final comment on the nature of organized dentistry will complete the background necessary for sympathetic understanding of the milieu of dental allied health education. American dentistry is a monolithic structure. All dentists belonging to the American Dental Association (ADA)—and most do—must belong to their local and state dental societies as well. Hence, the vast majority of dentists in the United States are bound by the rules and policies set by the House of Delegates of the national organization.

Governance of the ADA is, however, republican: members of the House of Delegates are elected at the state and local level. Therefore, as would be expected, the vast majority of the delegates are private practitioners and the policies set by the House, by and large, reflect the interests and motivations of the grass roots private practitioner. Policies governing actions of all Councils of the Association, including the Council on Dental Education and the Council on Dental Research, are determined by the House of Delegates. Thus the practicing arm of the profession utlimately determines the guidelines for the education of dentists and all dental auxiliaries, requirements to be met by their educational programs and the accreditation of all educational programs.

This operational structure has existed for many decades, and the House of Delegates of the ADA has come to view itself as the final authority in all matters related to the education and activities of dental manpower and in determining what research would be appropriate. Fortifying this presumption has been the fact that the Board of Dental Examiners of each state—which has purview over accreditation of educational programs at the state level, licensure of graduating dentists and dental hygienists, and the determination of activities permitted dental auxiliaries—is largely composed of dental practitioners who work in close cooperation with organized dentistry at the state and national levels.

Considering this structure, it is understandable that little that was contrary to the wishes of the practicing dentist has transpired in dental education and the education of dental auxiliaries. Thus, as recently as 1961, the House of Delegates saw nothing unusual about adopting a policy which gave its Council on Dental Education the power to disapprove or approve all research related to expanded use of dental auxiliaries and to specify that the results of any research should not yield anyone who might be considered a second level dentist.[3] Only in 1970 did the Association finally concede that

it was inappropriate to continue a national policy which de-
terred and prohibited research.[4]

Individuals from other walks of academic life may be surprised to learn that their colleagues in dental education have
tolerated such obviously flagrant infringements of the basic
tenets of academic freedom. Yet, in final analysis, this should
appear no more startling than other paradoxical aspects of
the field of oral health and its consignment to the backwaters
of human concern. Indeed, until there are substantial signals
that dental neglect is no longer to remain a national ethic,
there will continue to be some difficulty in separating fool-
hardy from heroic dental leadership.

Signs of Change

While many dentists in the United States may hope that the
nature of dentistry during the first half of the twentieth century will somehow be the nature of dentistry of tomorrow,
much is happening which makes this hope quite unrealistic.
These tides of change have great importance for the field of
dental auxiliary education because they challenge the authority of organized dentistry, especially as it relates to control of
dental auxiliaries and their education.

This past year the School of Dentistry at the University of
Kentucky tested and won a strong legal opinion supporting
the school's freedom to teach what it wished and to whom.
This landmark decision established that state boards of dental
examiners and state dental societies are no longer the final
authority concerning the content of dental education or dental auxiliary education. While similar legal controversies may
continue to arise, the ultimate outcome is obvious.

During 1972 the ADA learned that its existing system for
accreditation was not in line with new federal guidelines governing conflict of interest in matters of accreditation. Two
fundamental changes are required. First, the ADA House of
Delegates must relinquish its traditional role as final authority
in these matters. Second, laymen must be included among the
membership of future accrediting bodies to assure that public
as well as professional interests will be represented.

Also during 1972, pressure from the consumer movement resulted in the appointment of laymen to the Boards of Dental Examiners in several states. It seems reasonable to assume that this change will extend to all boards in the near future. As this occurs and as the role of consumer representatives on such boards takes firmer expression, the traditional coincidence of policy and interests between boards and state dental societies will disappear.

Finally, 1972 witnessed a major attack on the monolithic structure of the ADA in the form of a legal case challenging the requirements that a dentist must belong simultaneously to a local, state and national components. Regardless of the outcome, it is clear that the very existence of this challenge has irreversibly weakened the habit of conformity which until now has provided a unique strength to organized dentistry.

While several years will pass before the full impact of these changes will be felt, it is obvious that quite suddenly the dental practitioner and organized dentistry have lost absolute control over the important mechanisms by which the evolution of the profession and its auxiliaries have been controlled. In the future, the prerogatives of academic freedom, consumer interests and independent thought will increasingly color this control process and, as a consequence, it is to be anticipated that the pace of dentistry's evolution will be greatly accelerated. The transition from tortoise to hare is, however, not an easy one; it is to be hoped that new participants in the controlling mechanism will exert patience and restraint until the profession realizes that rather than having lost anything, it has in fact been given the opportunity to expand its horizons to the fullest.

Most would agree that 1972 presented dentistry with more than enough problems to digest for some time to come. Unfortunately, there are other items of equal concern on the agenda for the immediate future. All of these have a special relevance to the field of allied dental health because their successful solution would seem to necessitate the use of many more auxiliaries, perhaps with more sophisticated training programs.

The United States is the only advanced nation which has no

formal dental care program for its children. Legislation to bring such a program into being has been proposed in recent years and was again introduced in Congress for 1973. Were this program to be enacted and funded in adequate fashion it would thrust tens of millions of new young patients into a dental care delivery system which is already reasonably in balance with its patient load.

There is a very rapid expansion of dental care programs wherein a third party handles the arrangements and payment for care on behalf of beneficiaries. Fundamental to the success of these programs is the need for the third party to impose quality control procedures and continuously to seek maximum benefits from minimum cost. To date, the full impact of these two restraints has not been felt by the present dental care delivery system, but it is certain that when it is, the existing capacity of the system will shrink unless many more auxiliaries are employed.

The threat of alternate systems to the private practice system is also stimulating the dental profession to explore more fully new ways to provide more care of high quality for more people at lowest possible cost. An important facet of this challenge is the development of better ways to match the availability of dental care to the widespread nature of oral disease. Here again, the employment of greater numbers of auxiliaries seems to hold the key to both problems.

Thus, it is not surprising that much of the current activity of the dental profession is focused on a study of dental auxiliaries and dental auxiliary education in search of ways to mobilize both to help the profession cope with its problems. Not all of this effort is progressive, but this too is not surprising considering the nature of oral disease and the nature of dentistry. Moreover, the whole nation is presently in a love affair with the past and this mood is agreeable to a profession which still is better equipped to serve the "good old days," when excellent oral health was a luxury to be enjoyed by the few who could afford it. Eventually, unless there is a great depression, all eyes will again turn forward and this promises to be a time of rapid advancement for dental auxiliaries.

In the interim, the situation is most confusing. Progressive,

status quo and regressive plans and programs for dental auxiliaries are proliferating across the nation. Everyone is in the
act. Government, schools of dentistry, schools of dental
hygiene, schools of dental assisting, institutions of higher
education, dental societies, state boards of dentistry—as well
as the national associations of dentists, dental assistants and
dental hygienists—are all involved. But within each group
there is little consensus about the future roles of dental auxiliaries. This confused state of affairs would seem to be ample
justification for administrators of educational institutions to
take a hard look before approving the initiation of new programs for dental auxiliaries. Yet, there are a large number of
independent new programs in various stages of development,
particularly in the community college sector of higher education. This suggests a lack of awareness of several critical problems within the present system of dental care delivery. Either
those not yet involved know something that has escaped those
in the field or they are unaware of the following problems.

Major Items on the Agenda for Dental Auxiliary Education

Major problems in the field of dental auxiliary education can
be summarized in the form of a few pressing questions to
which there are at present no answers: What types of dental
auxiliaries will there be in the near future? What will each of
them do? Where, how, and for whom will they work? Where
will they be trained? How many will be needed? When will
they be needed? Who will teach them? How much will this
training cost? How much will they earn?

That these questions have no relation to the familiar dental
manpower arrangement which has existed for the past half
century illustrates the extent of the problem. Yet, these were
among the major questions being addressed by American
dentistry in 1972. On the basis of the information presented
so far, the reader should not be too surprised to find that
dentistry has gotten into such a quandary or that there is not
much definitive progress to be reported for the past year.
There were, however, some noteworthy events which, while

not providing answers, at least give some indication on the way matters are proceeding.

The Identity Crisis. Dental auxiliaries face a loss of their identity, and this is presenting dental auxiliary education with a problem which has few counterparts in the history of education. Quite literally, neither dental hygiene educators nor dental assisting educators any longer know with certainty what sort of graduate they should be producing by 1975. Three years ago no great uncertainty existed. Since the disappearance of definitive career objectives occurred so precipitously and the long-range implications are still largely unknown, there is quite naturally great concern among dental auxiliary educators regarding the future of their programs. Their concern is not the basic one of losing one's usefulness to society but rather a psychological one involving the prospect of forsaking a familiar identity for an as yet undefined new one.

The problem arose in the following fashion. Since the beginning of dental hygiene, the dental hygienist has been a licensed auxiliary. Each state established rules and regulations in its dental practice act governing the functions and duties for dental hygienists. As rules and regulations go, those devised for dental hygienists were the most restrictive ever imposed upon a health professional. Recalling the nature of the dental profession, it is understandable that dentists would have followed no other course with their first licensed auxiliary. Dental assistants, on the other hand, are not licensed and therefore their duties are not proscribed in dental practice acts.

Thus, when pressure to explore the expanded use of auxiliaries finally became irresistible during the sixties, two factors favored the selection of dental assistants over dental hygienists. First, there were no laws specifying what assistants could or could not do. Second, if dental hygienists were chosen, it would be necessary to change the law (i.e., dental practice act) in every one of the 50 states; nearly everyone considered this an unrealistic possibility. Therefore, on these practical grounds, the field of dental hygiene was put on ice for an entire decade, while the dental assistant or individuals with no prior dental training whatever were utilized in research directed at exploring expanded functions. Quite naturally this research, to be meaningful, included intraoral procedures, and the clear-cut line which had traditionally separated the dental assistant from the dental hygienist was obliterated.

This formed the basis for the current identity problem. Subsequent findings from the research further complicated matters because they did, indeed, show that bright young people could learn to perform many intraoral procedures without all the knowledge and skills of either the dentist or the dental hygienist. The identity problem was further exacerbated by tentative proposals for entirely new names for auxiliaries, such as dental therapist, oral therapist and assistant dentist.

During 1972 the House of Delegates of the American Dental Association endeavored in characteristic fashion to clarify the situation by passing a resolution to the effect that there are only three dental auxiliaries; namely, the dental hygienist, the dental assistant and the dental laboratory technician.[5] It will be recognized that such a pronoucement falls somewhat short of correcting the problem, but at least for the moment everybody knows who they are, if not what they are supposed to do.

The Facilities Problem. If clear heads and common sense could have held sway at the beginning of the sixties, the dental hygienist, for two very good reasons, would never have been excluded from the research which was probing expanded duties for dental auxiliaries. Dental hygiene has a well established curriculum possessing an extensive biodental component which is very suitable as an academic foundation for many expanded functions. Alvin Morris called attention to this asset during 1972 when he suggested that the dental hygienist should evolve into the assistant dentist of the future.[6] Of equal importance, dental hygiene schools possess the clincal facilities which lend themselves to the teaching of intraoral functions. Most schools of dental assisting fall far short in this regard, especially those which are separated from a dental school. Thus, the auxiliary which has been most favored for research related to expanded functions has, by and large, the least favorable educational environment in which to accomplish it.

Nevertheless, even though dental hygiene schools hold the advantage in respect to clinical facilities, a great many of them fall far short of being adequately equipped for the task of teaching extensively expanded functions. Hence, administrators of institutions of higher education who are contemplating modernizing the facilities of existing dental auxiliary programs or establishing facilities for new programs face a difficult decision. If they build in the image of the present, their facilities will be reasonably inexpensive, but they will probably become obsolete very quickly. If they build to anticipate the future task of teaching extensively expanded functions, the cost will be a great deal higher.

For example, a truly modern clinic setting adequate to teaching expanded functions related to restorative dentistry can run as high as $325,000 (exclusive of structure) for 15 teaching stations.[7] The reason for the marked difference in cost is, of course, that the educational environment required for the teaching of intraoral expanded functions differs little, if at all, from that of a dental school. Unfortunately, the current confusion over the future roles of dental auxiliaries has tended to keep this serious question from surfacing in discussions concerning the establishment of new dental auxiliary programs.

One solution suggested by Jerge in 1972 was for the dental schools to become dental manpower training centers.[8] Under this approach, auxiliaries trained in more modest satellite settings would be sent to the dental school for their final training in an advanced clinical setting. This suggestion does not seem to be widely applicable because the clinical teaching facilities for most dental schools are already overtaxed. In addition, there is the more general issue of whether dental auxiliary programs will be truly welcomed into the university environment or merely used as pawns in some bigger game.

The author painfully recalls that as a dean he awakened one morning just over a decade ago to find that his plans for his school to become a dental center devoted to training all types of dental manpower in a team situation had been skuttled. A university decision had severed affiliation with the one dental hygiene school in the area because, as a two-year program, it did not fit the university's image of what constituted higher education. This problem apparently is still current since a paper by Rovin suggests that even dental schools are not entirely comfortable within the fold.[9]

The Faculty Problem. Once the future role of dental assistants and dental hygienists has been settled, most of the faculties of dental schools will need additional training. During 1972 the U.S. Public Health Service began a program at its Louisville, Ky., installation for training dental auxiliary educators to meet expanded responsibilities. The emphasis is presently on preparing individuals to assist in the operation of the TEAM (Training in Expanded Auxiliary Management) programs in dental schools wherein dental students are given experience in managing groups of auxiliaries performing expanded functions.

If, however, the time comes when auxiliaries will be called upon to perform more advanced intraoral procedures, individuals possessing the dental degree will have to be added to the faculties of dental auxiliary schools on a full-time basis. This step is inevitable because, even when dental auxiliaries on the faculty become skilled in teaching these advanced procedures, a person with the dental degree and license must be present to assume responsibility for the welfare of the patient under treatment.

The introduction of the full-time dentist educator into the present system of dental auxiliary education will create serious difficulties. First, this step will skyrocket the cost of programs because at least two dentists must be on board to assure that at least one is in the clinic at all times. Since less than one out of five dental auxiliary programs is physically attached to a dental school, most schools are not even in a position to rely on a parent institution for emergency coverage. Second, dental auxiliary training programs, as Castaldi has pointed out,[10] tend to have small classes averaging only 19.5 students as compared to nursing schools, which average 29.4 students.

Therefore, it may well be financially unfeasible for many programs to carry the higher cost of teaching advanced expanded functions. Finally, small dental auxiliary training programs located in areas having a low density of dentists may not be able to attract dentist-educators at almost any price.

If one disregards temporarily the monumental problem of providing adequate experience in an actual clinical setting, a program initiated in 1972 promises to do much to help dental auxiliary educators to take on the responsibility of teaching expanded functions at the preclinical level. The program is called ACORDE and involves all the dental schools in the United States in a coordinated effort to develop a standardized self-instruction course in operative dentistry.[11] Progress to date suggests that it will be possible to deliver educational packages which will enable students working on their own with minimum guidance from instructors to fully prepare themselves for introduction to the clinical scene. The long-range significance of this program for dental auxiliary education, especially if similar programs related to other facets of dentistry are developed, is obvious. But it also highlights the need to find quickly some solution to the problem of adequate facilities for subsequent clinical instruction.

The Problem of Patient Supply. The training of dental auxiliaries learning to perform intraoral procedures ultimately involves a clinical setting having an adequate flow of patients. Yet, it is surprising how often this simple truth escapes the attention of both those advocating the establishment of new programs (dentists in the area) and those contemplating the move (the administrators of institutions).

In earlier times when dental health manpower was trained on the poor for practice on the rich, an adequate supply of patients was not much of a problem. Today, however, this approach is no longer tenable on moral, constitutional and practical grounds. Therefore, educational institutions must increasingly seek patients from the same pool being served by the dental practitioner. This is a relatively new situation and many dentists have yet to realize it is part of their responsibility as members of a health profession to relinquish patients to the educational system. They are more apt to view the efforts of educational institutions to recruit patients as being no different than the unethical solicitation of patients by one of their fellow practitioners. The friction has been further increased by the efforts of the dental schools to expand the experience of their students beyond the walls of the schools through programs involving them in care delivery situations within the community.

It is clear, therefore, that as dental auxiliary education moves in the direction of expanding the clinical training of its students, it will be creating additional stress on the patient pool and institutions should anticipate encountering at least some criticism from local practitioners. The conflict will be less in areas having an adequate population to meet the needs of the school without impinging unduly on the income of the dentists in the area. Hence, it would be prudent for institutions contemplating the establishment of new dental auxiliary schools to give careful thought to this matter, particularly if they are at all desirous of establishing schools which have the capacity to evolve into more complex educational programs lying over the horizon.

Frank prior discussions with the local and state dental societies concerning patient supply may help avoid the unpleasant situation whereby an institution's efforts to meet the obligations of providing adequate clinical experience for its students exposes the faculty to official criticism for having violated the Codes of Ethics of these societies. The author personally encountered this problem during 1972. The Codes of Ethics of the American Dental Association and most state dental societies evolved in a bygone era and consequently are primarily designed to govern the practice of dentistry. As a result, most codes do not address the needs of educational institutions and, if strictly interpreted, make no distinction between dental care delivered as a part of education from dental care delivered by practitioners. Failure to make such a distinction has the unhealthy effect of casting education as a competitor of practice.

The leaders of dental education in Massachusetts are currently working with the Dental Society to produce a modern

Table 1

Mean Income of Independent Dentist by
Number of Auxiliary Personnel (1970)

No. of positions (full time)	Mean net income
0	$19,333
1	24,249
2	32,684
3	41,547
4	45,030
5 or more	55,245

Code of Ethics which will address the special needs of educational institutions. It is hoped that a model code for the nation will result from this effort.

The Numbers Game. Those interested in a detailed and comprehensive statistical analysis portraying the employment of dental auxiliaries in the United States can obtain this information from the 1971 Survey of Dental Practice.[12] A few data, however, have been extracted and summarized in order to illustrate certain points and trends (see Tables 1 and 3).

From Table 1 it can be seen that it is in the dentists' self-interest to employ dental auxiliaries. Data illustrating this point began to appear over a decade ago and from the trends shown by Table 2 the point was not lost on the profession.[13] Since the number of dentists in 1971 only approximated the number of auxiliaries employed full time, it is clear that future employment prospects for additional auxiliaries are excellent from a nationwide viewpoint. However, the picture is often not so bright close to centers which educate auxiliaries. But from the data in Table 1 it would appear that dentists in areas having a scarcity of auxiliaries could well afford to help solve their problem by offering special salary incentives as an inducement. The average annual salaries paid to full-time auxiliaries in 1971 were: dental hygienists, $8,424; dental assistants, $4,764; and dental laboratory technicians, $8,436. Thus, a dentist working alone could offer a 25% incentive to a dental hygienist and a dental assistant and still raise his net

Table 2

*Estimated Number of Auxiliary Personnel
Employed by Independent Dentists*

	1962	1965	1971
Dental Hygienists (full time)	5,700	9,700	15,800
Dental Assistants (full time)	68,700	81,400	99,200
Dental Laboratory Technicians (full time)	3,100	4,300	4,900
Total full time	77,500	95,400	119,900
All Auxiliary Personnel (full and part time)	122,000	144,300	205,300

income from $19,333 to $29,387. This approach would seem more realistic than endeavoring to establish marginal dental auxiliary education programs in unfavorable environments.

Table 3 shows that there is a general similarity in the employment of auxiliaries nationwide. The data are presented, however, to serve as a reference against which to note that in one state which still recognizes apprenticeship training for dental hygienists (Alabama), more dentists employ a full-time hygienist (50.3%) than in any other state. Georgia, which recently abandoned apprenticeship training, has the second highest percentage (43.2%). The relatively high rate of employment of full-time dental hygienists in the Southeast, as shown in the Table, reflects Alabama and Georgia practice.

Other state dental societies have noted this phenomenon and during the past year a few have indicated interest in reinstituting the prerogative of apprenticeship training for dental hygiene. It should be noted, however, that formal dental hygiene education has not existed in Alabama for many years, which raises the question as to whether the two systems for training dental hygienists can coexist. While the American Dental Hygienists Association is no doubt aware of the seriousness of this threat to the very foundations of its profession, it is apparently under irresistible political pressure

Table 3

Percentage of Independent Dentists Employing
Auxiliary Personnel, by Region and Type of Personnel (1971)

	Dental Hygienist		Dental Assistant		Dental Laboratory Technician	
	Full Time	Part Time	Full Time	Part Time	Full Time	Part Time
New England	20.9	19.1	72.2	24.5	4.0	1.1
Middle East	14.9	12.8	66.5	21.7	2.9	1.3
Southeast	23.6	13.3	90.5	15.9	6.6	2.3
Southwest	12.4	11.3	89.7	19.7	6.6	3.3
Central	13.3	14.4	78.3	25.3	3.3	2.5
Northwest	16.0	10.8	85.4	21.7	6.6	2.4
Far West	13.2	23.9	86.2	21.2	4.8	1.9
United States	15.8	15.4	79.2	21.8	4.3	1.9

since its 1972 House of Delegates conceded that because of
"social pressure," revision of the traditional licensure requirements specifying that individuals must be graduates of
accredited educational programs is warranted.[14] Obviously,
every educator interested in formal dental hygiene education
should follow this apprenticeship question very closely.

It will be noted in Table 3 that in all regions about the same
percentage of dentists employ a part-time dental hygienist as
employ a full-time one. One reason for this, which explains
why dental hygiene is such an attractive career, is that dental
hygienists can earn a good income and be very helpful to a
dental practice even though they are involved only part time.
Consequently, many elect to work part time in order to enjoy
greater personal freedom.

The 50-State Maze. At the 1972 meeting of the House of Delegates of the American Dental Association the following resolution was adopted:[15]

Number 229, *Statement of Policy on Utilization of Dental Auxiliaries for
Expanded Duty Functions.* In the training, education and utilization of
dental auxiliaries for the purpose of assisting the dentist in providing high quality dental care through expanded functions, it shall be
the policy of the American Dental Association that expanded functions shall be performed under the direct supervision of the dentist

and that auxiliaries shall perform only those functions *as defined in state dental practice acts* for which they have had appropriate education and training.

(Note: emphasis added.)

In the face of this directive, institutions which are interested in making certain that their students are given an education which will not limit their personal freedom and career horizons, should endeavor to tailor their programs to encompass the maximum expansion of functions permitted by any of the dental practice acts of the 50 states. The alternate course of teaching to a common denominator, which satisfied the most restrictive dental practice acts, would obviously be unfair to students, because they would be unqualified in one or another skill if they moved from one state to another.

The matter, however, is not so easily solved. At the same session of the House, the following recommendation was also approved as a resolution:

Number 234, Recommendation 26: The profession, through its various agencies, should accelerate the training and use of expanded function auxiliary personnel *in accordance with* state dental practice acts.

(Note: emphasis added.)

Very clearly, the practicing arm of the profession considers the political question of states rights far more important than the future welfare of students enrolled in dental auxiliary programs. Reflecting on the nature of the profession, this self-centered attitude can be understood, if not condoned. But the end result is to force dental auxiliary educators into a most difficult situation where they have no recourse but to stand up and fight for the principle of academic freedom even though they know that in doing so they will probably cause great embarrassment for the profession they serve.

Earlier in this chapter reference was made to the landmark decision in Kentucky wherein the attorney general held that the dental society, the Board of Dental Examiners or any special interest group could not interfere with the dental school's right to teach and do research. Yet, as this is being

written, the State Board of Dental Examiners in Massachusetts has sent all dental schools in the state an opinion from
the attorney general to the effect that a course offered to
students of dental hygiene allowing them to "drill and cut
hard and soft tissue" would be in violation of the Massachusetts Dental Practice Act. In contrast to this restrictive
ruling, the School of Dental Hygiene at the University of
Maryland already requires each of its students to have performed three gingivectomies before graduation.

Common sense will eventually dictate that educational institutions will decide what they will teach dental auxiliaries
and each state will decide what portion of this education and
training may be utilized within their borders. The Council on
Dental Education of the ADA is, of course, fully aware of the
current unsatisfactory situation and anticipates that new educational standards for dental hygiene, dental assisting and
dental laboratory technology will be approved by the 1973
House of Delegates.[16]

Dangerous Ground. No evaluation of the current status of allied dental health in the United States would be complete
without reference to an auxiliary who does not exist in this
country but whose presence eight thousand miles away in the
small nation of New Zealand has sent shock waves throughout
the American dental profession. This auxiliary, the New Zealand dental nurse, is trained in a two-year post-high school
program. She works for the New Zealand government in
small clinics attached to elementary schools and provides, at
government expense, routine dental care for 95 percent of
the children from age 2½ through 13½. The dental nurse
practices under the general direction of a district dental officer who supervises the work of from 75 to 120 dental nurses.

Two thoughtful reports by Friedman[17] and Dunning[18] in
1972, based upon first-hand observation of the results of this
53-year old program, indicate quite clearly that it has been an
outstanding success in New Zealand. When the program
began in 1920, Friedman reports, it was necessary for the
dental nurses to extract 78.6 teeth for every 100 restorations
placed while today extractions have been reduced to 2.8 per

100 restorations. Approximately 75 percent of all decayed teeth in New Zealand children are restored, compared to less than 25 percent in American children. The difference, as Friedman suggests, is due to the fact that 95 percent of New Zealand children receive routine dental care while half of the children under the age of 15 in the United States have never been to a dentist.

While the New Zealand program is aimed at the children, the benefits extend to the adult population. Dunning notes that between 1950 and 1968 the number of denture wearers declined from 45 percent to 26 percent among persons 20 to 29 years of age and for the 30-39 age group the decrease was from 68 percent to 50 percent.

The New Zealand program is socialized dentistry and this naturally makes it quite unacceptable in a country founded on the principles of private enterprise. Nevertheless, the program is worthy of careful study because it represents one of the largest and longest experiments ever conducted to find out whether by treatment alone dental caries can be brought under control. The answer from New Zealand is: "yes, massive treatment can control tooth decay."

After 52 years, the New Zealand program has reached a steady state and therefore provides solid data whereby one can calculate what it would take in terms of manpower and dollars to do the job in the United States. This latter aspect is not frequently mentioned but it holds great meaning for those interested in projecting the costs of a children's dental health program for the United States and the role dental auxiliaries might play in such a program.

Dunning's paper provides us with the basic data for the manpower calculations. There are 1350 New Zealand Dental Nurses for a population of slightly less than 3,000,000. To keep the ranks filled they graduate 200 new dental nurses a year from three schools. There are 14 district dental officers assisted by one to two dental nurse supervisors. In fluoridated areas one dental nurse can handle 700 to 1000 children, while in non-fluoridated areas the ratio is one nurse to 500. Therefore, for the United States, which is about 50 percent fluoridated, a ratio of one to 750 would seem to be a very reasonable

Table 4

Projected Manpower and Costs for a New Zealand
Dental Nurse Program in United States

	Manpower Picture	Estimated Cost per unit/year	Estimated Cost per year
U. S. Population 3-17 years old	60,227,000	—	—
Dental Nurses (1/750 children)	80,303	$10,000	$803,030,000
Dental Officers (1/96 DNs)	836	30,000	25,080,000
Dental Nurse Supervisors (1.5/1 DO)	1,254	15,000	18,810,000
Graduates per year (1/6.75 DNs)	11,896	9,150*	108,848,400
Number schools required (3 for 200)	178	—	—
Overhead (60% of salaries)	—	—	508,152,000
Total			$1,463,920,400

Plus

Clinical Facilities† $45,000 x 80,303 = $3,613,635,000
Training Facilities† $45,000 x 11,896 = $535,320,000

*Assumed cost is: $2,700 1st year; $6,450 2nd year
†Structure and equipment at 1 to 2 cost ratio

projection. In Table 4 the manpower system of New Zealand
is extrapolated to the United States along with some broad
general assumptions by the author concerning costs.

The most important figure in Table 4 is 80,303, which
represents a solid, conservative estimate of the number of
individuals (dentist or expanded duty auxiliaries) required to
provide routine dental care for the population of the United
States age three through 17. This figure is only about 20,000
shy of the current number of practicing dentists in the nation
caring for the *entire population*. If Friedman's estimate that in
the United States less than 50 percent of the children age 15
have ever seen a dentist is reasonably accurate, and the unlikely assumption is made that all of the rest receive adequate
care, then the very best reflection from the mirror of New

Zealand is still a shortage in 1972 of 40,000 individuals to provide routine dental care for the children of the United States.

Data presented in a 1971 ADA report entitled *Dentistry in National Health Programs*[19] reveals that even under the best of circumstances (i.e., all federal man power programs operating in 1970 would be in full operation during the decade) there would not be 40,000 additional dentists until 1990 and additional dental hygienists would not reach that number until the same year. Of course, by then the number of children would be up by more than 10 million and the total population would have increased by 25 percent.

The second most important figure in Table 4 is the $9,150 estimated cost of training an auxiliary capable of performing most of the duties of a New Zealand Dental Nurse. This figure is about two times the current cost of training a dental hygienist, but from the data emerging from the expanded duty research project at the Forsyth Dental Center in Boston the cost seems to be headed toward this level.[20] Even there, however, the cost would be only one-fourth to one-fifth that necessary to fully train a dentist and then place him in a situation which confines him to performing the routine care provided by the New Zealand Dental Nurse.

The third figure of interest in Table 4 is the estimate of $3.6 billion required to provide school dental clinics for the nation. Dunning concludes that the dental clinics must be in the schools in order for the system to work and thereby forces the system into a socialized posture which will quite understandably provoke violent opposition from the American dental profession. While a sum of several billion dollars is large, it is, however, less than the sum already invested by dentists in clinical facilities. Hence, it might not be impractical to think that the private enterprise system might rise to the occasion of providing clinical facilities conveniently close to the schools.

Indeed, one major research program in the United States is preoccupied with exploring whether dental hygienists trained to perform routine restorative dentistry *under the direct supervision* of dentists can enable the private practice system to increase its efficiency to the point of being successfully com-

petitive with alternate systems.[21] During 1972 ten graduate
dental hygienists were trained and then given sufficient clinical experience to bring them to a maximum level of productivity while maintaining a high standard of performance. During
the next two years various combinations of these advanced
skilled hygienists with existing types of dental manpower will
be studied to ascertain what mix yields the most dental care of
high quality for the least cost and whether this excels the
productivity of an otpimum mix of conventional dental personnel. These findings will provide necessary input data for
computer-generated models of dental practice being prepared by Pelton, et al.[22]

Research of this type is expensive. The cost of the Forsyth
project is running $300,000 per year exclusive of overhead,
largely due to the payroll for the many individuals involved,
namely, 2.5 FTE (full-time equivalent) dentists, 10 FT (full-
time) dental hygienists, 12 FT dental assistants and one FT
project secretary. Yet, it is only from comprehensive research
projects of this kind that sound conclusions concerning the
value of advanced expanded functions for dental auxiliaries
can be derived. Until the results are in, everything will be
mere speculation. It is to the great credit of the Massachusetts
Dental Society and the Massachusetts State Board of Dental
Examiners that they have appreciated the value of such research and fostered the progress of the Forsyth project.

From this brief review it can be seen that the New Zealand
Dental Nurse concept portends both promise and trouble for
the field of dental auxiliary education. Calmly explored, it
might enable dental auxiliaries to help the private practice
system meet all of society's expectations of dentistry. Irration-
ally opposed, it could become a most destructive force.

Summary

The intent has been to provide the field of higher education
with preparation for a more knowledgeable, but not necessarily less hazardous, exploration of a very challenging facet of
allied health education. The nature of oral disease and dentistry have been reviewed as a background for understanding

the attitudes and behavior of the dental profession relative to their auxiliaries and dental auxiliary education. Recent important events and trends which are causing fundamental changes in the identity as well as the role of dental auxiliaries were then described in terms of their possible impact on dental auxiliary education.

NOTES

1. "Report of the Inter-Agency Committee on Dental Auxiliaries," *Journal, American Dental Association* 84 (May 1972):1025-1084.

2. J. C. Greene, "Dental Health Needs of the Nation," *JADA* 84 (May 1972):1073-1075.

3. *Transactions*, 1961 House of Delegates, *American Dental Association* 222.

4. *Transactions*, 1970 House of Delegates, *American Dental Association* 43: 438.

5. *Transactions*, 1972 House of Delegates, *American Dental Association*, Chicago, Illinois.

6. A. L. Morris, "Meeting dental health needs through dental education," *JADA* 84 (May 1972):1076-1079.

7. R. R. Lobene, Director of Dental Hygiene Expanded Duties Research Project, Forsyth Dental Center, Boston, Mass. Personal Communication March 1973.

8. C. R. Jerge, "Dental dean offers program for nation." *Report, The University of Connecticut Health Center, Farmington, Conn.* (November 1972), p. 1.

9. S. Rovin, "The Dental School in the Educational Continuum," *JADA* 84 (May 1972):1063-1067.

10. C. R. Castaldi, "Dental Auxiliaries: dentistry's dilemma," *JADA* 84 (May 1972):1080-1087.

11. ACORDE (A Consortium on Restorative Dentistry Education) Bruce H. Bell, Chairman and National Coordinator, College of Dentistry, University of Florida, Gainesville, Florida.

12. "The 1971 Survey of Dental Practice," Bureau of Economic Research and Statistics, American Dental Association, Chicago, Illinois.

13. Bureau of Economic Research and Statistics, American Dental Association, Chicago, Illinois.

14. *Transactions*, 1972 House of Delegates Resolution 65, American Dental Hygienists Association, Chicago, Illinois.

15. *Transactions*, 1972 House of Delegates, ADA, Chicago, Ill.

16. J. M. Coady, Assistant Executive Director, Education and Hospital, American Dental Association, Chicago, Illinois. Personal Communication, February 20, 1973.

17. J. W. Friedman, "The New Zealand School Dental Nurse Service: lesson in radical conservatism," *JADA* 85 (September 1972):609-617.

18. J. M. Dunning, "Deployment and control of dental auxiliaries in New Zealand and Australia," *JADA* 85 (September 1972):618-626.

19. "Dentistry in National Health Programs." 2. "The requirements for dental and dental auxiliary manpower," American Dental Association, Chicago, Illinois. (1971), pp. 29-55.

20. R. R. Lobene.

21. R. R. Lobene.

22. W. J. Pelton, J. B. Dilworth, G. A. Overstreet, and O. H. Embry, "Comparison of Computer-Generated Data with Actual Use of Therapists." *Journal of Dental Education* 30 (February 1973):21-25.

CLINICAL LABORATORY EDUCATION

Ruth M. French

Education preparing students for service in the clinical laboratory is increasingly subject to the same stresses and demands that are current in general education. Responsibility and accountability are among the demands of learners and the public alike. In the clinical laboratory, responsibility has a number of points of impact, all related to quality performance: to the patient and his physician; to the public; and to those who are being educated. Responsibility to the public is for quality of results, of performance, and of education, within reasonable limits of expenditures. Learners have the implied right, if not contract, to expect quality in their learning experiences. The accountability is seen in cost effectiveness of the laboratory data generated, and the teaching/learning accomplished in the clinical setting.

Career education, described by Marland as that which reduces the artificial "distinctions between academic and occupational learning programs, blending them to serve all learners at all levels of instruction in their quest for productive careers and rewarding lives" is becoming increasingly acceptable.[1] It poses a challenge to the entire educational enterprise to re-examine traditional beliefs, to loosen social constraints, and push against inhibitions everywhere in order to respond to social changes.[2] In allied health, the demand is for more professional practitioners who have learned to teach, and who view teaching as an extension of the professional service for which they were originally prepared. Career education encourages more use of the variety of modes of instruction which focus on the learner's, rather than the teacher's, activities.

IDENTIFICATION OF ROLES AND FUNCTIONS

A root cause of many of the problems encountered in both education and manpower utilization is the lack of definition of roles and functions of medical laboratory personnel. The term "role" is defined as the part an individual fills, and the term "functions" is defined as the clusters of tasks he performs in filling his role. A basic assumption is that competency in roles and functions is not automatically the product of a diploma or certificate on completion of an educational program. It is unlikely that many would say that the bachelor of science guarantees better skills, but Gambino assumes that this is the belief. He writes: "About a decade ago, the ASCP Board of Schools eliminated the three-year program for ASCP registration, and went to a four-year college degree program for medical technologists. At that time, I wrote to the Board to express my conviction that more college was not a guarantee of better lab work."[3]

One has to deduce that Gambino's definition of a medical technologist is that of "trained hands," and assumes little, if any, judgment or application of basic principles. It is of interest, perhaps, to note that the mandatory degree requirement as part of the agreement between hospital-based schools and their affiliating institutions went into effect in January, 1973. The shift to which Gambino refers was a requirement for three rather than two preparatory years in college.

Berg[4] and Illich[5] tend to support Gambino's thesis that there is too much blind faith in degrees or education *per se.* Studies of Minnesota laboratory personnel did demonstrate a significant correlation between education and performance,[6] as did the national study by the National Committee on Medical Technology Education.[7]

In the consideration of roles, one has to broaden the scope to include medical specialty education when that specialty is as dominant a force as pathology is to allied health in the clinical laboratory. Gilpatrick and Siefer's work in task analysis of the field of radiology supports this assumption.[8]

In *Abstract for Action*, the report of the National Commission for the Study of Nursing and Nursing Education, the director, Jerome Lysaught, raises an important point relative to role definition.[9] He stresses the need for bilateral rather than unilateral efforts because of the necessity for congruence of roles when more than one profession is involved. The roles of pathologist and medical technologist are intertwined; those of the medical laboratory technician and laboratory assistant are intertwined with that of the medical technologist. Thus, the best definitions of roles will be the result of joint efforts so that congruence in both concepts and practice will be assured.

An intriguing proposal is forwarded by Copeland when he says: "We need several additions to our already active plans for a career ladder in laboratory medicine, first the *technologist-clinician* (emphasis his) . . . and I would like to propose that the technologist-clinician is already a fact, although not recognized as such yet."[10] He does not define the technologist-clinician other than to cite examples of a blood bank technologist making recommendations and a well-known hematology technologist acting as a consultant.

The need for definition of roles and functions is not only important in manpower utilization; it is essential for planning educational programs if they are to be truly relevant and productive of the essential competencies—effectively orchestrating content, learning activities, and student abilities. The national survey of clinical and public health laboratories conducted by the American Society for Medical Technology, under a contract with the Center for Disease Control, provides a wealth of information obtained from a total of 12,296 laboratories. In summarizing the report, Drury points out: "The Census found that 75% of all laboratories had either an administrative technologist or laboratory manager, and 26% of the total of 129,847 technical personnel identified hold supervisory positions. . . . These statistics should draw continued emphasis not only for career potential for technical personnel, but also on the need for expansion of management training both during the pre-employment education and as a part of continuing education activity."[11]

It has been recognized that more such content should be included in medical technology education, but the dimensions of the need have not been so well documented before. If the results of the survey can be so useful in educational planning, how much more so would be a definitive task analysis with its resultant definition of roles and functions.

MANPOWER AND STUDENT POOL

Another revealing combination of data from the previously cited laboratory census is summarized by Drury:

. . . only 656, or 20% (of the laboratories) reported that they had at least one vacancy. The total vacancies reported were 5,231. It is granted that in the future there may be a need for an increase in the number of trained medical laboratory personnel. . . . However, the need for personnel and concomitant training programs now may not be as extensive as proposed by some.

These results indicate that the extent of career recruitment efforts be studied to avoid overproduction of technical personnel for whom few jobs are available. . . . In 1971, the Registry of Medical Technologists certified 3,630 graduates as MT(ASCP). When another 2,735 MLT(ASCP), CLA(ASCP), HT(ASCP), and CT(ASCP) are added, all vacancies could be filled, and this does not begin to count those certified by AMT or ISCLT, proprietary and trade schools, and those trained personnel leaving military service that year.[12]

Contrast these hard data with the estimate of the Department of Labor, Bureau of Labor Statistics, that in seven years there will be 12,000 to 19,000 openings a year, with a total need for 190,000 laboratory workers. John J. McHugh, Associate Director of Professional Education, Department of Health, New York, is the source of this prediction,[13] which appears high even granting expansion because of legislative trends in health care. McHugh further believes that more training programs are imminent, and that the Allied Health Professions Personnel Training Act and special training grants will support them. Federal support of allied health education has been threatened and its future is uncertain.

Educators have the immediate concern of students seeking admission to various programs. It is not news that, "Except for isolated regional and local instances of shortage of students, allied health programs throughout the country are oversubscribed and are feeling admissions pressures comparable to those of medical and dental schools."[14]

There are a number of plausible explanations for this state of affairs, but explanations are not solutions. The burden of selection of qualified students who may reasonably be expected to be productive, safe practitioners rests squarely on the schools. Heretofore, admissions criteria could be rather ill-defined, primarily subjective in nature, and only estimates of the applicants' potential. Now, we must be able to document our decision-making in this critical area.

Though most colleges and universities face a comparable problem in general admissions, it is not compounded by the responsibility of screening out those who are inappropriately endowed for a career in a vitally important health occupation. To meet this responsibility, the faculty of the Curriculum in Medical Laboratory Sciences, Schools of Associated Medical Sciences, University of Illinois at the Medical Center, developed a statement of criteria for selection with an interview schedule and a reference check-list based on the criteria to document recommendations for admission. The students admitted to the class beginning work in 1973 will be the first group with which the criteria may be tested by achievement in course work and performance on their first jobs.

The question of who is to control entry into fields where job opportunities are decreasing cannot be easily answered. Some institutions may expand enrollment unrealistically, rather than risk being accused of artificially controlling numbers of applicants for employment. One cannot deny the qualified student on the basis of lack of job opportunities—that is largely his risk to take. Society, through its tax-based support of education, may very well be the determinant of expansion vs. cutback.

EQUIVALENCY AND PROFICIENCY EXAMINATIONS

The debate in relation to equivalency and proficiency examinations is focused on the assumption that paper and pencil tests can measure performance and affective skills in addition to knowledge. In programs that devote significant portions of the learning experiences to actual performance, it seems inconsistent to assume that testing for knowledge will define performance competencies.

This is not to say that knowledge of principles and ability to interpret data to solve problems are not important, but does suggest the need for more widespread and better definitions of what constitutes proficiency. Sound definition of course content and learning experiences are essential if equivalency credits are to be granted. The benefits to the student or prospective employer are obvious.

The examinations now available have been useful, making a significant step forward in both the work and academic areas of clinical laboratory activities. They undoubtedly have stimulated thought and action that is consistent with the goals associated with efforts to improve career mobility. The statement by both Educational Testing Service (ETS)[15] and the National Committee for Careers in the Medical Laboratory[16] that "Proficiency tests now offer laboratory directors a means of measuring job-related skills and knowledge . . . " implies that one can determine cognitive, affective, and psychomotor skills by paper and pencil tests. The skills referred to in the statement do not have definition. If they are cognitive, then the statement is accurate. If they involve other skills, it could be misleading.

A major problem in implementing the use of equivalency examinations, in which candidates have the opportunity to demonstrate the knowledge and skills necessary for a given course, is forcefully brought out in the data given in a comprehensive review of medical technology education by Rausch and Karni.[17] The authors surveyed 671 institutions in an attempt to find out how many offered printed descriptions of professional courses and corresponding credit hours. They obtained responses from 630 schools (94% of those surveyed), of which 548 met the criteria for the study. The catalogs of only 71 (13%) of the institutions surveyed supplied this detailed information on course content and credit hours to be earned.

Rausch and Karni focus on the implication of this fact in relation to the students' progressing on to graduate study, but it is also significant that, without specified courses and credits, there is no uniform application of the equivalency concept. The equivalency examinations are offered by ETS in its College-Level Examination Program. The norming population was drawn from among medical technology students who had completed work in the subject content of the examinations. These examinations are expected to facilitate the medical laboratory technician's completion of the baccalaureate degree, building upon the associate degree.

In a memorandum to medical technology education coordinators, T. M. Peery, Chairman of the National Committee for Careers in the Medical Laboratory, writes, "we sincerely hope that your institution will consider granting credit for clinical chemistry, microbiology, hematology and/or immunohematology on the basis of these examinations."[18] It is of interest to note that, in the preliminary work developing the examinations, ETS staff had difficulty in identifying the courses because they were not included in college catalogs, making it necessary for staff to interview selected institutions. In general, faculty of schools of medical technology are receptive to the use of written equivalency examinations, but expect to supplement them with an "in house" companion performance evaluation.

ACCREDITATION

The "Study of Accreditation of Selected Health Educational Programs" sponsored by the National Commission on Accrediting, the American Medical Association, and the American Society of Allied Health Professions has resulted in a number of significant recommendations.[19] This study has led the three sponsoring groups to consider the development of a Joint Commission on Accreditation for Allied Health. The establishment of such a Commission will open a new chapter for education in allied health. The responsibility for accreditation will be more broadly based, with representation from all sectors of education involved.

Accreditation of Schools

After nearly 30 years in accrediting schools of medical technology, the Board of Schools of Medical Technology of the American Society of Clinical Pathologists (a standing committee of ASCP) was replaced in December, 1973, by a new agency. The National Accrediting Agency for Clinical Laboratory Sciences is not under the direction of the ASCP or the American Society for Medical Technology, though a number of its members are selected by the two societies because they are sponsoring organizations. The Agency is the outcome of agreements between presidential officers of ASCP and ASMT, and other selected representatives.

The creation of NAACLS was the product of several interacting forces: 1) The vision and dedication of the medical technologists and the pathologists who were the Agency's architects; 2) The strong stance of the ASMT leaders and House of Delegates that, as a mature profession, medical technology has the responsibility and right to speak for itself; 3) The U.S. Office of Education's vigorous application of criteria for recognition of accrediting agencies; 4) The recognition of the importance of input from non-medically related educators and the public; and 5) The need to avoid proliferation of accrediting agencies.

The NAACLS organizational structure is made up of a Review Board (policy-making body), supported by committees responsible for serving the needs of several groups, viz., medical technologists, medical laboratory technicians, certified laboratory assistants, histotechnologists, cytotechnologists, and blood bank technologists. The Review Board's membership now includes three medical technologists, three pathologists, a medical laboratory technician, a laboratory assistant, a technologist-supervisor, a laboratory director, a college educator, a community college educator, and two public representatives. Aside from its significance within the medical laboratory field, NAACLS is being looked upon as an example to be emulated by others. There is, therefore, more than the usual responsibility to be met in fulfilling its charge.

Progress is being made in the development of better standards for accreditation of educational programs in the clinical laboratory field. For example, the 1972 *Essentials for an Approved Educational Program for Medical Technologists* embody changes that address the inadequacies noted by Rausch and Karni.[20] The changes require: 1) More individualization of college/university-integrated programs; 2) Documented evidence of the affiliation agreement between the hospital-based program and the college or university affiliate(s); 3) Clearer definition of prerequisites; 4) Use of modern principles of education in curriculum design and implementation; 5) Deletion of passing the Board of Registry examination as a degree requirement; and 6) Periodic self-study.

Definitions of the roles and functions of the medical director, program director, and educational coordinator reflect the evolution of different organizational structures among the various types of schools. As might be expected, these Essentials have been greeted with responses ranging from anxiety to relief, depending on the character of the existing programs. The object of the changes is the maintenance of quality education with a minimum of arbitrary restrictions.

CERTIFICATION

Early in 1973, the National Institutes of Health contracted with the Institute of Public Administration of Washington, D.C., to conduct a study of the feasibility of establishing a national system of certification for health personnel. This system was to be "conceived as an umbrella which could provide coordination and direction of certification practices for selected health occupations through voluntary participation."[21] Among the issues to be explored by the study were certification of new occupational groups and specialties; improvement of examination development, administration, and financing; and bridging certifying and licensing practices. Allied health professional groups were involved "to obtain their reactions to the design and operation of such a national certification system." Preliminary IPA findings indicate that such a system is feasible.

There is an increasing effort to focus attention on credentialing of individuals as an alternative to accreditation of programs. This approach emphasizes performance on the job rather than how or where capabilities were developed. In *Current Status of Credentialing for Health Personnel*, Maryland Pennell writes:

We should keep in mind the health needs of the patient and our major concern is the provision of services for treatment of disease and maintenance of health. We wish to dissipate any uncertainty or apprehension about the qualifications of those persons who perform the needed functions . . . we also wish to ensure sufficient numbers of qualified workers who have available to them opportunities for geographic movement and career mobility. The credentialing process provides the necessary measure to attain these results.

This is the time when national standards for qualifying health practitioners should be developed to provide direction toward alleviation of career mobility barriers in the health field. The standards should allow maximum degree of movement within and between professions or disciplines, with appropriate minimum qualifications for initial entry into the work force. And lastly, measurement of competence to meet these standards should be developed and incorporated into the credentialing process—be it accreditation of educational programs, certification of qualified personnel by the profession, or licensure of individuals by a government agency.[22]

In 1971 the U.S. Supreme Court ruled that pre-employment examinations must be job-related. If they serve other purposes, such as aptitude or intelligence testing alone, or if a high school diploma is required, violation of the Civil Rights Act of 1964 and thus discrimination is involved. Commenting on this case, Barrett points out: "Another implication is that the abolishment of a high school diploma as a requirement for employment may have broken the stranglehold of certification of institutionalized schooling in the United States. In other words, the door may be opening for other, less traditional kinds of training and schooling."[23]

She concludes her interpretative report with the following observations: "History is filled with examples of men and women who rendered highly effective performances without the conventional badges of accomplishment in terms of certificates, diplomas, or degrees. Diplomas and tests are useful servants, but Congress has mandated that they are not to become masters of reality."

A philosophic consideration of the need for job relevance in service to both the individual and society is the thought-provoking article by Blank, "Degrees: Who Needs Them?"[24] Although her focus is on degrees, much that she writes can be applied to certificate-awarding programs as well. She establishes her thesis by stating that: "The current emphasis on college degrees is also subtly but irrevocably denigrating the actual and potential fulfillments inherent across a broad spectrum of work. In other words, we are by definition (rather than by analysis) establishing two kinds of work: work which is labeled 'better' by having a degree requirement tagged to it; and all other non-degree work which through this logic, becomes automatically 'low level' or 'dead end'. . . . Note please that we are talking of degrees, not educational content or skills."

Blank's proposal is that people "be sorted out through actual performance, which is a far different crucible from what is used in meting out degrees . . . degrees, after all, are made up of credits, not capacities." She strongly supports "credentialing by measures of competence, rather than by completion of an approved program." It seems more equitable and profitable to delineate essential components of competence in cognitive, affective, and skill-related domains, and then develop evaluation instruments to measure the individual's level of competence against externally-determined standards of performance. Those who are engaged in consideration of accrediting specialist programs are in a position to plow new ground by first recognizing that the specialist's knowledge and performance competencies can be developed by experience in non-traditional modes, i.e., outside structured accredited programs. This is particularly true when such development grows out of prior education in a general or related field.

The American Medical Association's Allied Medical Educa-

Table 1

Type of Program	Number Approved
Medical Technology	728
Medical Laboratory Technician	14*
Certified Laboratory Assistant	176
Histologic Technology	22†
Cytotechnology	110
Blood Bank	61

*Essentials approved in 1971; accreditation of programs in progress; approximately 200 in operation.
†Essentials approved in 1970; accreditation of programs in progress; many more in operation.

tion Directory, 1973, contains information that could lead to shifting attention to individual credentialing rather than program accreditation for specialty areas.[25] In March, 1974, the Allied Health Newsletter included the numbers of approved schools or programs in allied health professions and services. Table 1 shows the numbers of clinical laboratory-related programs currently approved.

It is obvious that the processing of applications for new programs and resurveys of accredited programs periodically constitutes an extremely heavy load, burdening volunteer personnel. Expert or near-expert surveyors are all too few as it is. The question that inevitably arises from these data is: with an already overloaded system, is it either wise or realistic to add more work? The objective of ensuring quality patient care is of unequivocal importance. However, adding work compounds existing problems; it could lead to half-way accomplishment of the objective and leave the validity of the accrediting system in question.

Unquestionably, a great deal of work would be involved in identifying essential components of competence and developing evaluation instruments. However, it should be less difficult to accomplish these two tasks when the field in question is relatively limited—as specialists such as clinical chemistry, microbiology, etc., are—compared to the medical technology generalist. In addition, it should be less difficult to obtain the necessary expert input for these tasks than to find willing volunteers, train them in survey techniques and judgment, and fund their survey visits.

The individual competency approach has the additional advantage of responding more readily to changing roles and functions and increments of new knowledge, thus fitting comfortably into periodic renewal of certification.[26] This sytem is being considered with increasing interest, and may well gain general acceptance. Both self-assessment and continuing education could be more productively used if essential competencies are identified. People can't perform to maximum effectiveness if they don't know what is expected of them and how they are doing relative to the expectations.

"There is a tide in the affairs of man which, taken at the flood, leads to fortune."[27] Now is the time. This is the tide.

CONTINUING EDUCATION

The importance of continuing education is well recognized. It is, in fact, a "big business," as reflected by the number of workshops offered in conjunction with national professional society meetings and at regional, state, and local levels. The Commission on Continuing Education of the American Society of Clinical Pathologists, according to Copeland, spends more than $1.5 million a year on this type of education—including publications, instructional materials and workshops.[28] In addition to its national meetings, the American Society for Medical Technology offers a variety of workshops at regional levels, providing opportunities for all types of laboratorians. The Society's self-assessment program is growing in content areas and participation.

The stimulus for all this activity is, of course, the surety that what is known and used today will be added to or modified, and that practitioners must adopt continuing education as a way of life if their competencies are to keep pace with developments and thus meet the demands of modern practice. A logical next step is to translate non-credit-bearing continuing education into some type of credits applicable to merit raises and/or promotions, or to academic credit. This also has implications for recertification.

In 1971, the president of ASMT appointed an *ad hoc* Committee on Continuing Competency, with the charge "to study the matter of continuing competency and means of acknowledging value obtained from participating in continuing education programs in ASMT." The Society's House of Delegates approved a position paper on continuing education in 1971 which was the product of a subcommittee of the Education Committee, and laid the groundwork for the follow-up work done by the *ad hoc* Committee.[29]

The report of the *ad hoc* Committee to the Board of Directors of ASMT in June, 1972, summarized the resources studied and questions addressed.[30] The Committee noted that the focus was on continuing education as an indication of *intent* to maintain or improve competence, since there are no established uniform standards of performance or competence as yet. The assumption is that participation in continuing education activities undoubtedly leads to improved practice by most persons. The Committee report concluded with a proposal for an ASMT Continuing Education Award Program. Definitions of continuing education activities and those eligible for recognition were included, covering a range allowing for various kinds of participation accessible to any practitioner.

The Continuing Education Unit definition developed by a task force of the National University Extension Association, viz., 10 contact hours "under responsible sponsorship, capable direction, and qualified instruction" has been adopted as the qualification for one CEU. The continuing education award program was endorsed by the ASMT House of Delegates in 1973, both in principle and budget. The program was implemented in January, 1974 as Professional Recognition of Continuing Education—P.A.C.E. The entire issue of *Cadence* (November-December 1973) was devoted to P.A.C.E.[31] A system of evaluating applications for awarding Continuing Education Units to workshops and other educational programs, and recording CEUs for subscribing members is in operation, with more than 2,000 members enlisting in the program to date. Non-member clinical laboratorians may also participate in the program for a nominal fee.

SUMMARY

As part of the fabric of the general American education enterprise, education for careers in clinical laboratory sciences is subject to the same critical analysis of goals and mechanisms for their achievement as is education in other fields. Consequently, there are pressures for implementation of accreditation that responds to public and student needs, competency-based curricula, continuing education programming, and competency-based credentialing. Significant progress is being made in accreditation, both as to the apparatus and the process. Positive responses are evident in designing competency-based curricula. Receptivity to systematic efforts toward competency-based credentialing is increasing. Opportunities for continuing education are growing at almost phenomenal rates, and mechanisms for appropriate recognition and use of participation are being developed. All of these elements create a climate of optimism which is essential to successful and continuing accomplishment.

NOTES

1. Sidney P. Marland, Jr., Foreword to *Essays on Career Education*, p. vii, published by Northwest Regional Educational Library, Portland, Oregon, under contract with the U.S. Office of Education/National Institute of Education.

2. *Report on Higher Education*, Department of Health, Education and Welfare, (Washington, D.C.: U.S. Government Printing Office, 1971), p. viii.

3. Raymond Gambino, "Deschooling the Laboratory," *Medical Laboratory Observer* (Sept. - Oct. 1972):113, 114.

4. I. Berg, *Education and Jobs: the Great Training Robbery* (New York: Praeger, 1970).

5. Ivan Illich, *Deschooling Society* (New York: Harper and Row, 1971), 1-15.

6. A. C. Kimball, H. Bauer, and V. Burres, "Blood Bank Procedures," *Minnesota Medicine* 47 (January 1964): 91-104; B. A. Merritt, R. B. McHugh, A. C. Kimball, and H. Bauer, "A Two-year Study of Clinical Chemistry Determinations in Minnesota Hospitals," *Minnesota Medicine* 48 (July 1965): 939-956; R. I. Heinemann, H. Bauer, and H. L. Knudsen, "Design for Development of Medical Laboratories: Personnel and Practices," *American Journal of Medical Technology* 25 (May-June 1959):145-165.

7. *National Correlations in Medical Technology Education*: A report of a study of medical technologists (Memphis, Tennessee: The National Council on Medical Technology Education, 1964), p. 6.

8. E. Gilpatrick and I. Siefer, *Health Services Mobility Study*, The Research Foundation of City University of New York (1971).

9. Jerome Lysaught, ed., *An Abstract for Action* (New York: McGraw-Hill Book Co., 1971), p. 88.

10. Bradley Copeland, "Future Shock—A Present Reality in Pathology," *American Journal of Clinical Pathology* 57, no. 6 (June 1972):699-714.

11. John Drury, "ASMT National Census Report," *Cadence* 4, no. 1 (January 1973):10-31.

12. MT—Medical Technologist; (ASCP)—certified by examination of the Board of Registry of the American Society of Clinical Pathologists; MLT—Medical Laboratory Technician; CLA—Certified Laboratory Assistant; HT—Histologic Technologist; CT—Cytotechnologist; AMT—American Medical Technologists; ISCLT—International Society of Clinical Laboratory Technologists.

13. "Medical Laboratory in 1980: New Job Titles and More Job Openings," news story reported in *Medical Laboratory* 9, no. 2 (February 1973):18.

14. *AAMC Weekly Report* 73 (20 February 1973):7.

15. *Bulletin of Information for Candidates*, Proficiency Examinations for Clinical Laboratory Personnel (Princeton, N.J.: Educational Testing Service, 1972-73).

16. *Proficiency Examinations for Clinical Laboratory Personnel*, Progress Report XII, 31 January 1973, Attachment B, "How to Use Proficiency Examination Results" (Bethesda, Md.: National Committee for Careers in the Medical Laboratory).

17. V. Rausch and K. Karni, "A Tilt at a Windmill?—A Study of Medical Technology Education," *American Journal of Medical Technology* 38, no. 6 (June 1972):216-228.

18. T. M. Peery, *Memorandum* (Bethesda, Md.: National Committee for Careers in the Medical Laboratory, 10 January 1972).

19. W. K. Selden, Director, Study of Accreditation of Selected Health Professions, *Part I, Staff Working Papers,* October 1971; *Part II, Staff Working Papers,* February 1972; and *Commission Report,* May 1972.

20. *Essentials for an Approved Educational Program for Medical Technologists*, approved by AMA December 1972, effective January 1973.

21. Department of Health, Education and Welfare news release, National Institutes of Health, 26 February 1973.

22. Maryland Pennell, *Current Status of Credentialing for Health Personnel* (Bethesda, Md.: Bureau of Health Manpower Education, Division of Allied Health Manpower, 1972).

23. Jeanne Barrett, "Require a High School Diploma and You May Be Breaking the Law," *Career Development* (Washington, D.C.: Human Service Press, University Research Corporation, 1972).

24. B. D. Blank, "Degrees: Who Needs Them?" *AAUP Bulletin*, (Autumn 1972):261-266.

25. "Medical Education in the United States, 1971-72," *Journal of the American Medical Association* 222 (20 November 1972(:8.

26. S. K. Bailey, "Career Education and Competency-based Credentialism," *Essays on Career Education*, p. 221.

27. William Shakespeare, *Julius Caesar*, Act IV, Sc. iii.

28. Bradley Copeland, "Future Shock—A Present Reality in Pathology" (see note number 10 above).

29. R. I. Heinemann, et al., "Continuing Education for Medical Technologists, A Position Paper," *American Journal of Medical Technology* 37 (April 1971):147-156.

30. *Report of the ad hoc Committee on Continuing Competency*, (R. I. Heinemann, Chairman), Board of Directors, American Society for Medical Technology, June 1972.

31. *Cadence* 4 (November-December 1973):6.

RADIOLOGIC TECHNOLOGY:

The Birth, Growing Pains & Maturing of a Profession

A. Bradley Soule

"A New Kind of Rays"

Radiologic technology as applied to medical science might be said to have begun at the University of Wurzburg, Germany, on November 8, 1895, when Wilhelm Conrad Röntgen made his epochal discovery "eine neue Art von Strahlen"—"a new kind of rays"—which he termed "x-rays."[1] One of the first x-ray photographs he made was a picture of the bones of his wife's hand. His observations were recorded in three classic reports in December, 1895, March, 1896, and May, 1897.

News of Röntgen's discovery was flashed around the world and the potentialities of this new modality in medical and surgical diagnosis were immediately recognized.

Almost anyone who had available the essentials for generation of x-rays—an electrostatic machine or an induction coil, a Crookes tube, a fluorescent screen and a few other pieces of equipment—hooked them up and started making x-ray exposures of anything available, including human bodies. Many of the early experimenters in this country were physicists because of the ready availability of equipment and their scientific knowledge and interests.

The first documented medical x-ray examination in North America was performed at Dartmouth Medical School on February 3, 1896, by Edwin Brant Frost, professor of astronomy, assisted by C. F. Emerson, professor of physics. The patient was a 15-year-old boy who had sustained a fall several weeks before, injuring his forearm.

The x-ray examination, performed with a Crookes tube energized by an induction coil, entailed an exposure of 20 minutes and the developed plate clearly demonstrated a fracture of the ulna.

An enterprising photographer, possibly with a sense of the historic significance of the event, captured the scene. This photograph and a print of the roentgenogram are displayed today with understandable pride in the lobby of the Mary Hitchcock Memorial Hospital in Hanover, part of the Dartmouth-Hitchcock medical complex.

So great was the interest in the scientific world—and among the public at large—that scores of people scouted around to find equipment with which to generate these new rays: the early months of 1896 showed use of x-ray by at least 50 scientists, including Thomas A. Edison.

Soon physicians and medical students and many others had joined the ranks. The pioneers were a motley lot, also including pharmacists, dentists, photographers and just plain gadgeteers of all ages. In many respects the latter resembled the people, many of them quite youthful, who a generation later were the radio buffs who sat up until the wee hours of the morning tinkering with home-made crystal sets trying to tune in Station KDKA in Pittsburgh or WBZ in Springfield.

The ardor of many of these early workers was soon dampened by the realization that x-ray was a two-edged sword which damaged tissue even as it produced valuable information hitherto unobtainable.[2]

During 1896, very serious "burns" were encountered by many of the early workers. As the risks became apparent, greater precautions were taken. In 1902, Dr. E. A. Codman of Harvard Medical School reviewed all papers on x-ray injuries that he could find in both the European and American literature and could locate less than 200 cases.[3]

The "burns" led to painful ulcerations which would not heal, and many of those affected were subjected to a series of amputations and skin grafts. In a high percentage of cases, malignancy supervened and the victims died, hardly beyond the prime of life.

However, the injurious effects of x-rays were soon exploited by applying them in the treatment of cancer. Dr. E. H. Grubbe of Chicago claimed to have used x-ray in the treatment of a patient with carcinoma of the breast on January 29, 1896.

THE EARLY DAYS: EACH X-RAY SPECIALIST HIS OWN TECHNICIAN

One of the pioneers in the diagnostic field was Walter James Dodd, Chief Apothecary at the Massachusetts General Hospital in Boston who, with the collaboration of his assistant, Joseph Godsoe, constructed an x-ray machine in the hospital and began producing roentgenograms of patients and also performing fluoroscopy. This met with enthusiastic response on the part of the medical staff and Dodd and Godsoe found themselves devoting most of their time to this fascinating new tool. Needless to say, they were both badly burned by the damaging rays and Dodd died about 20 years later as a result of malignancy incurred from exposure of his hands and face.

It soon became evident to Dodd that this new modality was to play an increasing role in medicine, so that in 1900 he entered Harvard Medical School. He stayed but one year since his knowledge of x-ray was so sought after that he could not devote the time necessary for study of medicine in Boston. He then enrolled in the University of Vermont in Burlington where he completed his medical studies in 1908. Throughout this period of about twelve years he was the "x-ray specialist" at the Massachusetts General and, while in Burlington, would make weekend trips to Boston to interpret the radiographic plates and to perform fluoroscopic examinations.

Another near-pioneer was Dr. Paul C. Hodges. In an engaging autobiographical sketch, "A Radiological Odyssey," published in condensed form in the January, 1973, issue of *The Pharos*,[4] Hodges, now emeritus professor of radiology at the University of Chicago, tells of working as a 15-year-old boy in an x-ray laboratory run by his uncle with equipment dating back to 1898. Now 81 and nearly as active as ever in scholarly and investigative work at the University of Florida, he later earned his way through medical school at the University of Wisconsin by taking and interpreting x-rays at the University Hospital, where he was proud to be the "x-ray man."

Within a year of Röntgen's discovery, young Walter B. Cannon, later the famous physiologist, then a freshman medical student at Harvard, rigged up an x-ray machine and fed bismuth and barium preparations to cats, geese and other animals and made tracings of his fluoroscopic observations on toilet paper, thus initiating gastro-intestinal roentgenology.

During the succeeding years, physicians gradually took over the use of x-ray and soon it was apparent that emerging was a new medical specialty of roentgenology. Most of these x-ray specialists performed their own examinations and this practice persisted well up into the twenties and thirties. A number of them engaged young men and women as apprentices and taught them how to position patients, make x-ray exposures and develop the plates.

Ed. Jerman, Radiologic Technology's First Teacher. One such layman, Ed. C. Jerman, realized that these technical workers were invaluable members of the x-ray team. Employed as an engineer by General Electric Company, Jerman was among the first in the country to produce roentgenograms (January, 1896). He soon began instructing pupils in the art of radiography, thus providing the beginnings of formal training in this field. He was instrumental in bringing about the creation of the American Registry of X-ray Technicians (ARXT) in 1920 and joined the Board as Examiner in 1924. His book, *Modern X-ray Technic*[5] was about all the technical literature then available to the novice technician or to the physician entering the field. Models of clarity, Jerman's books are prized today as invaluable mementoes of the period.

The Registry Board[6] was sponsored originally by the Radiological Society of North America and the American Roentgen Ray Society, the latter withdrawing its support in 1927. The Board evaluated candidates on the basis of rather meager credentials and by written examinations, largely based on Jerman's books. Shortly thereafter, the technicians formed the American Association of Radiological Technicians (later, the American Society of X-ray Technicians)[7] and in 1926 voted to accept only *registered* technicians as members. By 1927, 432 candidates had qualified.[8]

During the next decade, the x-ray technician had established himself as an indispensable aid to the roentgenologist. During the twenties, thirties and even well up into the forties and fifties, many were trained informally. This meant that while they were working under the supervision of a radiologist in a hospital or office, a considerable number received no formal instruction and were literally self-trained.

Largely due to the influence of Jerman and a number of teaching-oriented radiologists and technicians, training programs were developed, mainly in large metropolitan hospitals associated with medical schools. Most of these were one year in length and placed the greatest emphasis on the practical aspects of training.

In 1936, the Registry Board established a list of approved programs based on a survey of medical schools and hospitals and by 1943 there were 150 on the "approved" list. To make it independent of registration, accreditation was later transferred to the American Medical Association which, through its Council on Medical Education and Hospitals drew up *Essentials for an Approved School of X-ray Technology* and set up a plan for inspection and accreditation of schools. The minimal acceptable program was one year in length, with a basic minimum curriculum of required subjects and hours. In 1943, the American College of Radiology superceded the RSNA in assuming joint sponsorship of the Registry with the American Society of X-ray Technicians, and this arrangement has been in effect ever since.

Alfred B. Greene and his Influence on Education, Accreditation and Registration. In 1933, at about the time Ed. Jerman dropped out of the picture, a bright young x-ray technician who had been "curing" for tuberculosis and working at the Glen Lake Sanitorium in Minnesota, took over the part-time direction of the activities of the Registry. Alfred B. Greene, a graduate of the University of Minnesota and a registered technician, thus started a brilliant career which lasted until his retirement in 1965. In 1942, the office of the Registry was moved to Minneapolis and Greene assumed the position of Executive Secretary of the Registry Board.

In this crucial period and the years that followed, Al Greene's influence was stronger than that of any other person in pointing out the path which technology was to take in what has since been referred to as "The Golden Age of Radiology." He was also active in the American Society of X-ray Technicians (ASXT) and served as secretary-treasurer, editor of the journal, *The X-Ray Technician* (now *Radiologic Technology*) and, later, as president.

Three years after his retirement in 1965, the Registry Board established in his honor the Alfred B. Greene Program in Continuing Education for the purpose of advancing the careers of teaching and administrative technologists. The Program supports ARRT-sponsored courses at universities.

For a time, staff inspectors of the AMA conducted survey-inspections of training programs of radiologic technology. These were frequently perfunctory visits made by physicians often inexperienced in the problems of education of technicians. Many of the programs offered little more than an apprentice type of training.

The Struggle for Recognition and Better Education

During the 1950s and early 1960s, efforts to improve the quality of educational programs were intensified largely through the intelligent and determined efforts of a group of talented leaders in the American Society of X-ray Technicians (ASXT), including members of the Education Committee. Many of these had come up the hard way through apprentice training and were keenly aware of the needs for higher standards of education, accreditation and registration.

Some of the names that stand out among scores of others are Clark R. Warren, Richard A. Olden, John B. Cahoon, Erminda R. Clark, Martha G. Hampel, Marjorie C. Tolan, Ralph J. Bannister, Theodore T. Ott, Dante DiLella, Leslie Wilson, Robert L. Coyle, Neil J. Lyons, Jean A. Widger, Robert I. Phillips, George Koenig, Mary L. Rudder, William Raymond MacInniss, Eileen McCullough, Edward W. White, Meredith G. Lewis, Patricia O. Mueller, and of course Al Greene and his successor, Roland C. McGowan. A few of these have disappeared from the scene but most of them were quite young at the time and are still active.

The ferment had strong grassroots support from many of the technicians in the field. It came at a time when hundreds of new schools were being developed throughout the country to meet the rapidly increasing demands for more and more trained workers in the field. A true missionary spirit prevailed which has persisted to this date.

The principal objective of the ASXT was to raise educational standards by developing improved instructional programs, not only for staff x-ray technicians but also for teaching and supervisory personnel.

Radiologist trustees serving on the Registry Board, most of them dedicated and interested radiologists and experienced teachers themselves, were of inestimable help. They presented the technicians' plight and objectives to the American College of Radiology[9] and the Council on Medical Education of the AMA and obtained their support.[10]

During the same period, one of the successful devices developed to improve technician-radiologist relationships was the introduction of "off-the-cuff" informal get-togethers held at the time of the annual meetings of the ASXT and attended by the officers and trustees and committee chairmen of the Society and by the trustees of the Registry Board and the Committee on Technologist Affairs of the College. Here the technicians could present not only their gripes and grievances but also their hopes, aspirations and recommendations to the representatives of organized radiology. These sessions produced an upsurge in interest on the part of the Board of Chancellors and Councilors of the College and, through them, of the members.

Largely as a result of these and other meetings, steps were taken to elevate standards of education and accreditation. The school inspection program was taken over from the AMA by the Councilors of the American College of Radiology, who performed the inspections at their own expense.

Another major accomplishment was the revision in 1960 of the AMA *Essentials of an Accredited School* which established the two-year program as a minimum standard for training. Educational programs in nuclear medicine and radiation therapy technology were created and encouragement was given to the development of college-affiliated programs, chiefly with junior colleges but with some universities as well. These were designed to produce teaching and supervisory personnel, which were in extremely short supply.

Technicians who had long aspired to professional status were dignified by being named "technologists." The Registry became the American Registry of Radiologic Technologists and the Society became the American Society of Radiologic Technologists. Work began on programs to train and certify technologists in the specialties of Radiation Therapy and Nuclear Medicine. The first examinations in Nuclear Medicine Technology were given by the ARRT in 1963 and in Radiation Therapy Technology in 1964.

The problems of how to handle the weak schools was a knotty one. The instructors in most of these had come up through the ranks with little or no formal training. Schools were needed, however, not only because of the amazing proliferation in numbers and types of radiologic examinations being performed but also by the fact that technologists trained in metropolitan teaching centers were frequently loathe to seek employment in rural and semi-rural areas.

The Commission on Technologist Affairs responded by developing a new inspection program in which a technologist experienced in teaching and supervision joined the radiologist as a member of the survey team. If weaknesses or deficiencies were uncovered through inspection the program was required to correct them before being granted approval. The inspecting team also served in an advisory capacity which, in most instances, was greatly appreciated by those running the programs. This team approach was successful in raising the educational standards and in stimulating school directors to strive for excellence in their programs.

The Education Committee of the ASRT developed an excellent Teachers Syllabus[11] designed in "cookbook" style to follow the Basic Minimum Curriculum. Twice revised, it offers a complete outline of each of the required and most of the elective courses, fairly explicit instructions on how to teach radiologic technology, and a compendium of teaching aids to help the teacher in presentation of material.

Refresher courses for all levels of technologists were offered at national and regional meetings and institutes were held annually in different parts of the country with especial emphasis laid on the offering of educational material directed toward the needs of teaching and supervisory personnel.

The Junior College Enters the Health Professions Field. The remarkable proliferation of junior colleges in the country played its part in the development of training programs in radiologic technology. For a number of years associate degree programs had been offered in a few community colleges, chiefly in California; the basic didactic instruction was provided in the colleges and the practicum in radiology departments of cooperating hospitals. However, during the middle and latter sixties, nearly 1,000 colleges appeared on the academic scene, many of them offering low or free tuition to residents of the areas and offering a wide variety of opportunities for education, not only in general fields but also in vocational areas.[12] More and more began to include radiologic technology and its subspecialties. This came at a time when hospitals were overburdened with costs of educational programs and relief in payment of faculty salaries in schools of nursing and technology was welcome. The junior colleges provided the didactic instruction; the hospitals, the practicum.

Guidelines were established by the ACR Commission on Technologist Affairs, and the responsibilities of the educational institution and the cooperating hospital or hospitals were spelled out after much time, thought and agonizing. A shortage of qualified teachers oriented to the needs of students training for various types of clinical practice was offset, in part, by the decidedly higher level of academic competence in the college faculty than in many of the hospital-based certificate programs.

The NACOR Report. The second major factor in boosting demands for more skilled professionals in the field of radiology was the publication in April 1966 of the third in a series of reports of the National Advisory Committee on Radiation (NACOR).[13] The report traced the remarkable growth in the health professions and called attention to increasingly severe shortages of manpower in all branches of the radiologic sciences.

Not only were radiologists in short supply but there were also gaps in: (a) non-physician professional personnel, including radiological engineers, radiochemists, radiological physicists, radiobiologists and radiological health specialists; (b) technical personnel, including clinical x-ray, radiation therapy and nuclear medicine technologists and technicians; and (c) other supporting personnel, including nurses and administrative staff.

In October, 1967, the Medical X-ray Advisory Committee to the Surgeon General of the Public Health Service (PHS) identified four major groups of technologists and technicians in short supply:[14] (a) senior technologists instructors; (b) general purpose technologists; (c) highly specialized specific purpose technologists; and (d) limited purpose technical personnel with short training.

Growth and changes in the types of radiologic services were produced by the increase in number of diagnostic procedures per hospital admission from 1.50 in 1946 to 4.42 in 1961.[15] Advanced and complex new techniques in diagnosing and treating cardiovascular and cerebrovascular abnormalities, utilization of artificial body parts, transplants of organs and various electronic devices and prostheses all established the performance of highly complex and time-consuming radiologic procedures requiring the services of specially trained radiologists and supporting personnel. Most of these were in short supply.

In 1967 there were approximately 72,000 people operating x-ray equipment in the country.[16] Of these, approximately 33,000 were qualified (registered) technologists working in all phases of x-ray technology. Hospitals employed 24,000 technologists, 84 percent being full-time and 16 percent nonregistered, either full-time or part-time.

The PHS estimated that by 1975 100,000 technologists

would be needed, at least 52,000 of them fully trained.

Of 49,000 registrants of the ARRT in 1967, it was estimated that approximately one-third were not actively engaged in professional practice.[17] Seventy-three percent of this third were women, most of whom remained active for only one or two years after training. The paucity of males reflected the field's lack of attraction for the young man who contemplates supporting a family in the nation's inflated economy. Low salary scales had long been traditional in the field, without any effective ladder which might permit a technologist to advance his responsibilities and income.

Of the approximately 5,000 graduates of schools of radiologic technology in 1967, 99 percent came from hospital-based schools with so-called "terminal" programs which did not qualify students or graduates for college credit. About 50 received associate degrees and only 13 obtained baccalaureate degrees.

The National Conference on X-ray Technician Training. Largely as a result of these reports, the Division of Radiologic Health of the Public Health Service organized a National Conference on X-ray Technician Training. Meeting in September, 1966, at College Park, Maryland, 350 people gathered to consider the question: "What will it take to provide adequate numbers of qualified operators of x-ray machines in medicine?" Those attending included officers and members of the Commission on Technologist Affairs of the ACR, and of the ARRT and ASRT, technologist teachers and supervisors, physicists, radiobiologists, representatives of industry and labor, public health officials and others. The published report of the Conference details the findings, which indicated a serious shortage of radiologic personnel at all levels and offered suggestions for developing and implementing educational programs designed to produce more radiologists, radiation and health physicists, radiobiologists and technical workers.[18] Basic weaknesses in the then current system were deficiencies in training programs; an alarmingly high drop-out rate; low salary levels unattractive to men; little opportunities for advancement; lack of a career ladder with relative absence of middle management types of position; need for more and better teachers and administrators.

Numerous suggestions came out of the conference, including direct attack on these weaknesses. It was suggested that not only should the 24-month hospital-based programs be continued and upgraded but a better organized system of postgraduate studies and of university and college programs directed toward the education of administrative and teaching technologists should be encouraged and supported. Greater recognition of the technologist and commensurate implementation of salary levels and development of a career ladder should be made more available, in the hope of attracting more qualified applicants for training and of assuring them of opportunities for advancement. It was emphasized that fully trained technologists are needed as much in rural areas, smaller hospitals and doctors' offices as in larger urban settings; that a patient should not be penalized with second-rate care because of his geographic location.

Other conclusions: 1) While the basic 24-month, hospital-based program should be, at least quantitatively, the backbone of the training effort, these should be improved and expanded and new programs developed where needed.

2) Innovative programs in such areas as "radiologists' assistants," radiology department administration, and others should be explored and encouraged if found promising.

3) Federal support through the USPHS should be encouraged, including a grants program under which qualified and promising educational programs could be subsidized, at least in part, to support faculty positions, to provide students' stipends or scholarships, to improve physical facilities such as libraries, study areas and classrooms where needed, to provide audiovisual aids, etc.

4) Postgraduate and refresher courses should be developed, particularly for technologists already in the field, on such subjects as teaching and administrative methods and techniques, recent advances in radiologic and business equipment and instrumentation, principles of radiation protection, programmed learning methods, equipment maintenance, etc.

5) Efforts should be made to bring inactive technologists back into the field, possibly starting with a pilot study to determine the potential for recruitment of technologists and for development of refresher courses for them. Subsidization of technologists and of schools might be required during periods of retraining.

The ferment which resulted from this Conference stimulated all groups concerned with educational programs in radiologic technology to increased activity.

The Joint Review Committee on Education in Radiologic Technology. The AMA Council has been for a number of years the organization recognized by the U.S. Commissioner of Education as the responsible accrediting agency for educational programs for specific health disciplines, including radiologic technology. The Council has sought to establish and maintain standards of quality for educational programs and to provide recognition of those which meet the standards established and to encourage and assist in the development of new programs.

In 1962, there were 718 AMA-approved programs of radiologic technology, five in junior colleges and two offering a baccalaureate degree. In 1972, there were 988 hospital certificate programs and 125 college programs, 20 of which offered baccalaureate degrees. The college-affiliated programs utilized 582 hospitals for the clinical practicum. Thus in 1972, there was a total of 1,554 clinical facilities involved in the training of radiologic technologists (Table 1). By February 9, 1973, 16 new college programs were pending, awaiting survey inspections and Board action.[19]

Ground rules for educational institutions providing instruction in radiologic technology were amended and the corporate structure of organizations concerned in planning, inspection and accreditation came in for extensive review.

The role of supervising the inspection of schools previously handled by the Committee on Technologist Training of the ACR was taken over by a new Joint Review Committee on Education in Radiologic Technology,[20] sponsored by the ACR and ASRT.

Table 1

Radiologic Technology:
Comparative Statistics of Schools,
Students, Graduates and Registrants by Specialty

	1952	1957	1962	1967	1972
Total No. of AMA Approved Schools of Radiologic Technology	310	517	718	1,047	1,113
Schools with Less than Two Year Program	187	164	26	0	0
Two Year Programs	122	350	685	1,004	988
Associate Degree Programs, 2-2 1/2 Years Each	0	2	5	39	105*
Baccalaureate Programs	1	1	2	4	20*
Total Clinical Facilities Involved	310	522	720	1,100	1,554
Total Student Capacity	2,200	3,974	7,739	14,214	19,021
Total Graduates	1,080	1,966	2,315	4,939	6,661
Enrollment	1,907	3,212	6,231	13,335	17,816
Total Graduates from Associate Degree Programs	0	15†	26	102	250†
Total Graduates from Baccalaureate Programs	—	—	—	13	40†
Total Registered Technologists (ARRT)	11,000†	18,000†	31,000†	49,000†	72,000†
Total Inactive RTs	—	—	—	17,000	—
Total Registered Nuclear Medicine Technologists (ARRT)	—	—	—	400	1,940
Total Registered Nuclear Medicine Technologists (ASCP)	—	—	—	—	339
Total Registered Radiation Therapy Technologists	—	—	—	180	600

*Involving 582 hospital radiology departments
†Approximate

The Committee examines applications and records of educational programs and reviews the performance of graduates; it requests site evaluations when indicated, reviews the survey reports and makes recommendations to the AMA Council on Medical Education as to approval status. It also acts in an advisory capacity to institutions initiating new programs and works to improve the quality of existing programs.

CURRENT EDUCATIONAL STANDARDS

Radiologic Technology. The *Essentials of an Accredited Educational Program for Radiologic Technologists* were last revised by the House of Delegates of the American Medical Association in December 1969.[21] These provide, as in the past, that acceptable schools may be conducted by approved medical schools, radiology departments affiliated with accredited general hospitals or by accredited institutions of higher education which have clinical affiliations with approved medical schools or radiology departments affiliated with general hospitals.

While the major emphasis on instruction is in the area of diagnostic roentgenology, including some of the more complex radiologic procedures, some instruction must be provided in nuclear medicine and radiation therapy technology.

The directing radiologist must be eligible for certification by, or have been certified by, the American Board of Radiology or have qualifications acceptable to the Council on Medical Education of the AMA.

There should be at least one instructor who is a trained radiological technologist, registered or eligible for registration by the ARRT, who may serve as assistant director of the school, assisted by a corps of well trained technologists. There must be at least one qualified technologist instructor for each three students.

The educational program must comprise a minimum of 24 months including 410 or more hours of didactic courses and adequate clinical experience in a hospital department. The course should follow a planned outline similar to the *Curriculum and Teacher's Syllabus in Radiologic Technology*. The new

Essentials also require that degree granting programs must conform to the guidelines established by the ACR Commission on Technologist Affairs. These guidelines spell out in some detail the requirements which must be met by the degree granting institution and by the cooperating radiology departments. In essence, the responsibility of each Associate Degree Program in Radiologic Technology is vested in the institution awarding the degree. Whereas the integrated clinical experience is inherent to the hospital radiology department, the contractual arrangements between the two institutions should clearly define the responsibilities and obligations of each.

Two categories of associate degree programs are acceptable for evaluation for approval: (a) junior colleges without campus-based energized radiological laboratories; and (b) junior colleges with campus-based energized radiological laboratories and teaching aids designed to simulate the clinical environment insofar as possible and acceptable to the radiologist-technologist directors responsible for coordination of the training program.

The ACR guidelines offer detailed suggestions for curriculum with both required and elective courses offered in four college semesters.

Also stipulated is a minimum of 2,400 hours of hospital clinical experience (not including the didactic 410 hours professional major) in those degree programs without campus-based radiological laboratories. A reduction of hospital clinical experience (not including the 410 hours of professional major) to a minimum of 2200 hours is considered adequate for those programs having campus-based energized laboratories.

It was noted that most such programs will require more than 24 months for completion but that each must be evaluated on its own merit to validate compliance with the stated minimums.

Copies of these *Essentials* and those on Radiation Therapy and Nuclear Medicine Technology may be obtained from the Joint Review Committee on Education in Radiologic Technology.

While the guidelines were designed principally for junior (or community) colleges, a number of universities have developed both associate and baccalaureate degree programs in radiologic technology.

Attempts have been made in a number of educational institutions to assure students of both lateral and upward mobility. At the University of Vermont, a School of Allied Health Sciences has been organized with certain courses shared during the first year with students enrolled in the two-year program in radiologic technology, technical nursing and medical laboratory technology. All rad-tech students take the same basic courses during the first year but follow separate curricula during the second year in either diagnostic x-ray, nuclear medicine or radiation therapy technology.

Of the 35 students in the entering class, 25 are enrolled in diagnostic x-ray and five each in radiation therapy and nuclear medicine. If a student's interest changes, he may apply for transfer to one of the other categories or to one of the other programs in the School of Allied Health Sciences; this may be accomplished if an opening exists.

At UVM, a student may continue on to receive a baccalaureate degree if he or she qualifies academically, but in one of the other colleges of the university. Under study is a proposed BS program in radiologic technology, to be completed in eight semesters plus required practicum in the affiliated hospital radiology department.

The total length of time required for the present associate degree program in radiologic technology varies with different students who must complete 2200 hours of practicum. Some elect to use summer vacation time for part of this and some prefer to follow it with an extended practicum in the affiliated hospital department.

Radiation Therapy Technology. As early as 1960, the ARRT with the cooperation of the ACR Committee on Radiation Therapy Technologist Training Programs started planning for certification of people in the specialty of Radiation Therapy. The first examination in radiation therapy technology was given in 1964.

In December, 1968, the House of Delegates of the AMA approved the first *Essentials of an Acceptable School of Radiation Therapy Technology*, prepared by the AMA Council on Medical Education with the cooperation of the ACR, the ARRT and the ASRT.[22] In essence, this established a required twelve-month course of training in radiation therapy either in an approved medical school or in the radiology department of an accredited general hospital. The course of training was to be given in a complete radiation therapy department conforming to *Guides for Determining Standards of Radiotherapy in Major Cancer Management Centers*.

It was designed to be presented in approximately 260 teaching hours and followed a planned outline similar to the curriculum designed by the ASRT and the ACR Committee on Radiation Therapy Technologist Training Programs. Didactic instruction was to be supplemented by laboratory experience and daily clinical participation in the care of patients in the department.

Within a year, thirteen schools were recommended for approval and by January 1, 1973, thirty-three programs in Radiation Therapy Technology had been approved by the AMA Council.

Meanwhile, studies were under way to provide a satisfactory training program for technologists in the radiation therapy field within a period of two calendar years.

This culminated in December 1972 when the AMA House of Delegates approved a new *Essentials of an Approved Educational Program for Radiation Therapy Technologists—Two Year Program*,[23] produced by the same agencies which had developed the first *Essentials*. This provides for a broad-based educational program which might be conducted either by medical schools, junior or senior colleges or universities as well as by accredited general hospitals. The clinical phase of the educational program must be conducted in a major cancer management center which meets the standards set by the ACR.

These new *Essentials*, which will become operative and binding for approval of Radiation Therapy Technology Educational Programs, were to go into effect on July 1, 1974.

Nuclear Medicine Technology. The use of radionuclides in medicine for both diagnostic and therapeutic use began shortly after World War II. While most of these were initiated in departments of radiology, the development of more and more examinations involving clinical laboratory procedures engaged the interests of clinical pathologists and the increasingly wide applications of studies involving radionuclides brought many other physicians, chiefly internists, into the field, thus stimulating the development of the new specialty of nuclear medicine.

By 1960, work had begun on programs to train and certify people in Nuclear Medicine Technology. The ARRT gave its first examinations in Nuclear Medicine Technology in 1963 and by 1972 had certified 1,940.

The American Society of Clinical Pathologists, with the cooperation of the American Society of Medical Technologists, had been certifying medical technologists for many years. In 1964 it initiated a program for certifying nuclear medicine technologists and by 1973 had certified 339, chiefly medical technologists. The ASCP would accept candidates with either a high school diploma plus six years of on-the-job-training, or two years of college and four years experience.

A prolonged study then ensued sponsored by the AMA Council on Medical Education and involving representatives of the Society of Nuclear Medicine, the ACR Commission on Technologist Affairs, the American Society of Clinical Pathologists, the ASRT and ARRT, the Society of Nuclear Medicine Technologists and others, with the objective of establishing suitable standards for educational programs in nuclear medicine technology. These culminated in development of *Essentials of an Accredited Educational Program in Nuclear Medicine Technology,* which was given the seal of approval by the AMA House of Delegates in July 1969.[24] Under these *Essentials,* educational programs in nuclear medicine technology are accredited by a Board of Schools responsible to the Council on Medical Education of the AMA including representatives of the American College of Radiology, the Society of Nuclear Medicine, the American Society of Radiologic Technologists and the Society of Nuclear Medicine Technologists.

The Board of Schools is concerned with evaluation and survey of educational programs for nuclear medicine technologists and technicians, the maintenance of high standards of education and the development of new teaching programs.

Much credit is due Earle M. Chapman, M.D., for his skilled efforts as chairman of the Ad Hoc Committee of the AMA Council on Medical Education in bringing about the development of this new educational program and in developing the concept of the Board of Schools. The Executive Committee of the Society of Nuclear Medical Technologists selected Dr. Chapman as the first recipient of the SNMT Award of Recognition, for his contributions in advancing the professional excellence of Nuclear Medical Technology.

All candidates for admission to the program must have successfully completed four years of high school or have passed a standard equivalency examination for admission to college.

For the baccalaureate degree program designed to produce "technologists," three years (90 semester hours) of acceptable college credit with major in the biological or physical sciences must be supplemented by a twelve-month training program in an AMA-approved school of nuclear medicine technology. A registrant must have also qualified as a medical technologist—M.T. (ASCP), as a radiologic technologist—R.T. (ARRT) or as a registered nurse—R.N.

The associate degree program designed to turn out "technicians," requires successful completion of two years of study including a twelve-month training program in an AMA-approved school of nuclear medicine technology.

SASHEP

As noted, the Council on Medical Education of the AMA has been for many years the organization recognized by the U.S. Commissioner of Education as the responsible accrediting agency for educational programs for specific health disciplines, including radiologic technology in its various branches. The Council has sought to establish and maintain standards of quality for educational programs, to provide recognition of those which meet the standards established, and to encourage and assist development of new programs.

That the process of accreditation of educational programs and certification of workers in the allied health professions may be coming in for rather extensive overhauling was brought out in May, 1972, when a study commission developed to study accreditation of selected health education programs published the report usually referred to as SASHEP.[25]

The initiative for this study came from the AMA Council on Medical Education, acting upon recommendation of its Advisory Committee on Education for the Allied Health Professions and Services. Joining forces with the Association of Schools of Allied Health Professions and the National Commission on Accrediting, the sponsoring agencies developed the Study with support from the Commonwealth Fund.

Recognizing that accreditation of a number of health professions as they now exist has been in general a valued and acknowledged means of identifying educational programs of acceptable quality, the system has not been immune from increasing public scrutiny and criticism, both from without and within.

The Study Commission was developed in an effort to identify strengths and weaknesses in the accreditation of 15 health professional fields, and the Commission addressed itself toward offering possible new approaches in some or all of the areas.

The fourteen members of the Commission chosen to conduct this study were distinguished educators, all long-known and recognized for their experience and percipience in health-related professions. They were aided in their study by an equally able panel of advisors and by a full-time staff.

The report attempts to identify the issues involved in accreditation, certification, licensure and registration and probes deeply into many factors involved in such matters as accountability, structure, financing, expansion and research in these areas and their relationship to licensure and certification.

The report notes the remarkable proliferation of nonphysician personnel involved in the provision of health care during the past two decades.

The Commission considered and presented at least eight alternatives for the current method of accreditation. In its conclusions, it offered specific recommendations for the creation of a new organization under which accreditation should be coordinated, monitored and supervised by a national independent body governed by a policy board composed primarily of individuals who represent the public interest and also including individuals who may be directly associated with institutions, their programs of study, the professions, and the civil government.

Special cognizance was given not only to control over policies, criteria for recognition, procedures and practices of all current programs, but also to the initiation or extension of accreditation to include additional programs of study or new types of institutions in the health care field.

In this brief commentary, it is not feasible to attempt even to outline the many facets of this truly remarkable report. The reader is urged to obtain a copy for his own perusal from SASHEP, Suite 300, One Dupont Circle, Washington, D.C. 20036. (One copy free; additional copies one dollar apiece.)

The factual information derived and the recommendations which came from the Study will undoubtedly have far-reaching effects on accreditation of educational programs in the health profession areas and on certification of workers produced by these programs.

INNOVATIVE EDUCATIONAL PROGRAMS IN RADIOLOGIC TECHNOLOGY

During the past few years, a number of innovative programs designed to help meet the needs for specialized technical and administrative personnel have been developed in a number of university medical centers about the country. These have been designed primarily to produce different levels of professional competence, to provide a career ladder which might permit promising candidates to attain wider opportunities for advancement, and to break down the barriers which have existed in the past for most radiologic technologists. Many received grant support from federal agencies, and the Bureau of Radiological Health of the PHS was helpful in this regard.

During much of the period that followed the NACOR report in 1966, Arve H. Dahl, long a commissioned officer in the PHS and an engineer by profession, served as Director of the Office of Training and Grants. He immediately immersed himself in a study of the needs for personnel at all levels of radiological health. He soon became well-known nationally for his understanding of the nation's potential for producing such specialists as radiological and health physicists at the graduate and technician levels and of the calibre of training available in colleges and universities of the country.

He also sensed the need for more and better educational programs for radiological technologists and was instrumental in much of the planning that went into the Conferences on Technician Training and on College Affiliated Programs in Radiologic Technology described above.

Although handicapped by the exigencies of a limited budget for support of training projects, Arve Dahl had an almost uncanny ability to sense the potentials of innovative programs. Then with the aid of an able staff and an Advisory Committee consisting of concerned leaders in the fields of public health, health physics and education in the health sciences, he sifted out the less promising projects and enlisted the support of the Bureau for those that offered the greater opportunities for success.

Arve Dahl has retired, but his influence will long be felt for his contributions to radiological health in the United States.

University of Cincinnati Programs. One of the most comprehensive multi-purpose programs has been under way at the University of Cincinnati Medical Center. It involves both nuclear medicine technology and the development of radiology department administrators.

Nuclear Medicine Technology.
The first comprehensive degree-associated programs in the United States in the field of nuclear medicine technology were

developed at the University of Cincinnati by James G.
Kereiakes, Ph.D., and his associates, in the 1960s.

These programs, supported by training grants from the
Bureau of Radiological Health, PHS, have embraced the
fields of nuclear medicine physics and radiation health
physics as well as nuclear medicine technology.

Two programs were developed: a baccalaureate program
designed to produce "technologists" and a two year associate
degree program designed to produce "technicians."[26]

The baccalaureate program was set up as an option to the
existing four-year medical technology program already in
existence at the University of Cincinnati—the first two years
being identical to the medical technology curriculum. The
third year, however, was changed significantly, being directed
toward nuclear medicine technology. The fourth year consists of a 12-month internship in the radio-isotope laboratory of Cincinnati Medical Center and is largely of a practical
nature, including, however, a number of didactic lectures
designed to make the practicum more meaningful.

The two-year associate degree program provides a one-year
core curriculum in English, Psychology, General Chemistry,
Anatomy and Physiology and Mathematics, provided at the
Junior College of the University of Cincinnati. The second
year is almost identical to the fourth year internship of the
baccalaureate program, except that a few of the didactic sessions are omitted.

The nuclear medicine technology programs rely heavily on
material assembled and provided by the Technical Education
Research Center (TERC), Cambridge, Massachusetts,[27] the
Nuclear Medicine Subcommittee of the ACR Commission on
Technologist Affairs and the Joint Review Committee on
Educational Programs in Nuclear Medicine Technology.
TERC's searching and comprehensive studies were sup-
ported by a grant from the U.S. Office of Education, Depart-
ment of Health, Education, and Welfare.

In implementing these studies, a career ladder was developed, based in part on the Job Descriptions defined by the
ACR and ASRT.

The TERC group had estimated demands to prepare about

1,300 people for work in this field each year. It was also estimated that by 1980 approximately 16,000 nuclear medicine technologists and technicians would be required to serve the needs of the country.

Of Cincinnati's two programs, the baccalaureate was the first developed and by April 1974, a total of 21 people had graduated as nuclear medical technologists. Most of them are employed in supervisory, administrative and teaching positions in large nuclear medicine laboratories where their job performance has been rated as excellent. The associate degree program developed in 1969, had, by April 1974, graduated 14 medical radio-isotope technicians.

Members of the University of Cincinnati group believe that graduates of the baccalaureate program receive sufficient breadth and depth of knowledge to enable them to serve as chief technologists in a busy nuclear medicine laboratory or as instructors in the practicum of educational programs in the field. They feel that technicians trained in two-year programs will perform most of the clinical nuclear medicine procedures, and that the demand for technicians may be greater than for technologists by as much as three or four to one. They believe that student enrollment should be encouraged, especially in the two-year programs.

In February 1969, a colloquium on nuclear medicine technology training was held at the University of Cincinnati under the joint sponsorship of the PHS Bureau of Radiological Health and the Radioisotope Laboratory of the University. The published proceedings[28] provide much valuable information to those conducting or planning future programs at all levels in nuclear medicine technology.

Currently, there are in the country approximately 108 programs, 85 of which are certificate, 16 associate and seven baccalaureate. Others are in various stages of development and certification.

The "Rad-Ad" Project at University of Cincinnati.
In 1968, the University of Cincinnati initiated a graduate program in the field of health management designed to produce radiologic administrators (rad-ads).[29] The purpose was

to produce a high echelon worker who could relieve the radiologist-director of a department of many administrative details and assist him in the supervision and management of departmental activities.

Funded in part by a grant from the PHS Bureau of Radiological Health, the 15-month program is conducted at the master's degree level and comprises three quarters of classroom study, preceded and followed by one quarter of applied research and on-the-job experience. The didactic area embraces three major fields: Radiology, Public Health and Management.

The goals of the program are tailored closely to the needs of a segment of aspiring technologists and provide an incentive for the pursuit of advanced education. Most students, upon completion of the program, have been employed at salaries ranging from $12,000 to $16,000 with accompanying prestige inherent in a new professional niche.

The skills and knowledge developed in a talented technologist so trained offer promise for benefits to the patient, the technologist, the radiologist and the hospital administrative staff.

The training program was the subject of a symposium held in Cincinnati on May 22, 1970.[30] The basic discussion topics included prior training and experience necessary for success in the program, functions of radiologic administrators in hospital departments of radiology and critique of the prototype program. Also considered were potential sources of students, levels of instruction, placement of graduates, employment potentials and professional recognition of radiologic administrators.

Physicians' Assistants in Diagnostic Radiology: The University of Kentucky Study. One of the new experimental programs in radiologic technology is that designed to produce what have been referred to as "Physicians' Assistants in Diagnostic Radiology."

Campbell, Tuddenham, and others have demonstrated that it is possible to train radiologic technologists or even individuals without previous relevant training to screen specific types of diagnostic radiologic examinations, such as barium enemas, mammograms or chest roentgenograms, and to identify the positive from the negative studies.[31]

The objective is to determine the feasibility of training promising candidates from the field of radiologic technology to learn to perform as many duties as can be safely and appropriately delegated to them, while assuring that essential supervision and responsibility will remain with properly qualified radiologists. One such program was developed at the College of Medicine, University of Kentucky, several years ago, with grant support from the National Center for Health Services Research and Development, Health Services and Mental Health Administration, PHS.[32]

Students were trained to assist the radiologist in departmental administration, to perform fluoroscopic gastrointestinal examinations (these being taped for subsequent staff review), to aid in angiographic studies and to train other personnel to perform tasks that improve the radiologist's efficiency—such as coding diagnoses, arranging films on multiviewers—with particular emphasis on differentiating normal from abnormal roentgenograms. Instruction and experience also enabled the student to determine from an examination of the patient, his chart and radiographs the optimal roentgen studies needed to solve the patient's problem.

A three-year program was developed, two in the parent institution and one in a nearby medical facility.

During the first two years, two hours of didactic instructions were provided each day plus a considerable amount of individualized tutoring since the students arrive with different funds of knowledge and experience. The remainder of each day was spent in clinical rotations through such areas as intravenous urography, pediatric radiology, special procedures, nuclear medicine, gastrointestinal fluoroscopy and quality control—all under careful staff supervision.

Each student was assigned one rotation each year in the radiology department of another local medical institution where he gained experience in performing his duties in environments other than a university setting.

Evaluation begins with the administration of a battery of

tests upon admission to define his personal characteristics and aptitudes.

Each student agrees to accept employment for a year upon completion of the training program as a working physician's assistant in diagnostic radiology in a local medical facility in order to assess the quality of his professional labors and the level of acceptance he achieves from patients, referring physicians and the radiologic staff.

No data are yet available on these matters. However, this group of students averaged almost ten years of experience (two are required for admission) and all left positions of considerable responsibility.

At the University of Kentucky, a major effort of the program has been to train students to screen carefully selected radiographs for presence or absence of disease. Performance effectiveness is assessed from a consideration of percentage rates of false positive and false negative responses. The former are not a hazard to the patient since all false positives are reviewed by a radiologist, but they are, of course, inefficient. False negatives introduce a risk, since patients may leave the medical care environment under the incorrect impression that no disease exists.

Since even the most competent radiologists have been shown in numerous studies to make both false positive and false negative responses, the University of Kentucky investigators enlisted the aid of other groups to take the test examinations. These groups included staff radiologists, residents in radiology, medical students and radiologic technologists without training in this specialty, both at Kentucky and in several other university departments in the United States and Canada. Comparative test results showed that the University of Kentucky advanced radiologic technologist trainees did as well as most staff radiologists and decidedly better than most of the first-, second-, and third-year residents in both false positive and false negative interpretations.

The performance of students to date has exceeded the expectations of the staff, and unfavorable evaluations have been rare.

After what is admittedly a relatively short period of experience with this program, it is the considered opinion of those administering it and evaluating the work of the trainees, that selected radiologic technologists with appropriate additional training can safely and efficiently discharge many duties previously solely within the purview of physician radiologists. It is realized that it is necessary to confirm these data by showing that proficiency of this level continues and can be duplicated by successive groups of trainees.

It is not felt by the staff of the Department of Diagnostic Radiology of the University of Kentucky that physicians' assistants can in any way replace physician radiologists. If successful, however, the possibility of becoming a physician's assistant in Diagnostic Radiology will make a career in Radiologic Technology more appealing, since a new avenue for advancement will be available.

Other vexing problems, many of which are common to all types of physicians' assistants, remain to be resolved before physicians' assistants in Diagnostic Radiology can be utilized optimally in the delivery of radiologic care. It is held by some that the shortage of radiologists will disappear soon while others maintain a great need remains, particularly in academic radiology and in rural and ghetto areas. It seemed apparent to Mr. Huber in his thought-provoking article, that physicians' assistants in Diagnostic Radiology, particularly if it is shown they can accurately screen radiographs for the presence or absence of significant pathology, will contribute measurably toward increasing the pool of manpower to provide radiologic services.

The Physicians' Assistant in Radiology–the Duke Experience. The physicians' assistant program formulated by Duke University Medical Center has been training such personnel since 1965 to assume some of the duties heretofore relegated to the physician. Initially directed toward training helpers for those in general practice, it later was expanded to such fields as surgery, pathology and radiology.[33]

The pilot two-year program for physicians' assistants in radiology was initiated in 1969 by the Veterans' Administration in conjunction with the Department of Radiology of

Duke University Medical Center and with support from a grant from the Department of Education, Veterans' Administration, Washington, D.C. The first nine months was the same as that provided for other physicians' assistants but the remaining fifteen months instruction was similar to the University of Kentucky program.

Following completion of the program by the first three candidates, their performances and capabilities were evaluated carefully, both objectively and subjectively.[34] The critiques indicated that these hand-picked and unusually capable radiologic technologists were superior to special procedures radiologic technologists and their performance in the areas tested showed that they compared favorably with radiologists. All evaluators felt that the training had been highly effective.

It was the feeling of the Duke group that longterm analyses of the performance of physicians' assistants in actual work settings will be necessary before any final impression can be established as to feasibility, usefulness and acceptability of radiology assistants.

It was believed that the facilities and resources of Duke University Medical Center could best be utilized by concentrating on the development of a graduate level program in Radiologic Technology open only to registered radiologic technologists and designed to prepare students for positions such as supervisors, administrators, technical directors and special procedures technologists in the field of Radiologic Technology.[35]

Consequently, the long-standing and prestigious hospital-based two-year program and the Duke-Elon baccalaureate program in radiologic technology are being phased out and will be replaced by the new graduate level programs under development.

The Colorado Plan. Noting that the quality of training programs for radiologic technologists in hospital-based schools has been declining, largely because the programs have emphasized on-the-job training and have failed to make use of educational opportunities, Dr. Hendee and his associates developed what has become known as "The Colorado Plan."[36] Observing that the certificate programs contributed to low salaries and lack of professional recognition, with consequent imposition of limitations on vertical and horizontal mobility, a group of physicians, physicists and technologists explored the possibility of developing collaborative efforts with the University of Colorado School of Medicine and the Community College of Denver. Fourteen Denver hospitals with facilities for diagnostic radiology, nuclear medicine and radiation therapy were brought into the program in order to provide the greater part of the clinical practicum.

The first venture was in the development of an associate's degree two-year program. The Community College, supported by the State of Colorado and chartered to award the associate degree, provided a core curriculum for first-year students. Students could elect either diagnostic radiology, nuclear medicine or radiation therapy. Those who elected diagnostic radiology would continue to receive specialized courses at the college but would devote the major portion of their time in the radiology departments of the cooperating Denver hospitals to fulfill the required 2,200 hours of clinical training. Second-year students in nuclear medicine or radiation therapy technology would complete their training at the School of Medicine of the University of Colorado.

Upon completion of their training in any of the three curricula, graduates would receive the degree of Associate in Science and would be eligible to take the ARRT examinations in whichever field they were trained. All educational institutions were required to meet the qualifications of the Joint Review Committees on Educational Programs in Radiologic Technology and in Nuclear Medicine for approval by the AMA Council on Medical Education. A student capacity of 135 is listed by the AMA Council for the total program.

The Denver Collaborative Training Program is administered by an advisory committee comprised of physicians, physicists, technologists and educators from institutions participating in the program.

The programs in nuclear medicine and radiation therapy technology were supported in part for three years by the

Regional Medical Program of the PHS. This has now run out and the programs are functioning well with only minimal grant support.

The Policy Committee is now considering adding a program designed to produce technologists in the field of diagnostic ultra-sound. A junior-senior level program in health sciences administration has been established at Metropolitan State College in Denver; under study is the establishment of a similar program in health sciences education at the University of Northern Colorado in Greeley.

After three years, most of the graduates in all programs are employed in their fields. Several are continuing their education as full-time or part-time students at the University of Colorado or at Metropolitan, thus taking advantage of the career ladder which is an integral part of the Denver Collaborative Plan.

Radiology Aides–The Vermont Experience. Manpower studies in the field of radiologic technology noted the shortage not only of administrative teaching and special procedures personnel but also of lower echelon workers who can carry out easily learned tasks, thus relieving more highly skilled professionals of performing certain duties of a routine nature.[37]

In the School of Radiologic Technology of the Medical Center Hospital of Vermont, an experimental educational program was recently developed in the Department of Radiology of the University of Vermont College of Medicine, the aim of which was to produce "radiology aides."[38]

Many radiology departments have employed nontechnical and nonprofessional personnel, training them informally to perform certain tasks.

In Vermont, an attempt was first made to determine whether or not there was a place for a formal training course for such workers; how it would be structured; whether radiology aides so trained would perform a useful function in a hospital radiology department; whether they would be employable.

Encouraged by the results of these studies, a six-month training program was developed, largely financed by aid from the state office of the Manpower Development and Training Act (MDTA).[39] It provided reimbursement for instructional materials, instructional and educational counseling, supervision of didactic and practical experience, testing and evaluation, space and equipment used and instructional services, as well as monthly stipends and other allowances for students.

Selection of trainees was carried out through the usual Employment Service channels with supplementary screening interviews by the hospital departmental supervisory staff. For the first class of 15, trainees were selected from culturally and educationally disadvantaged healthy men and women between the ages of 17 and 55 years who demonstrated at least average learning ability on the basis of selected scores on the General Aptitude Test Battery. High school dropouts provided about half of the class.

Students were taught to assist in the performance of all types of radiologic examinations but *they were not taught nor were they permitted to administer ionizing radiation*. They transported patients to and from the department, placed patients on radiographic or fluoroscopic tables, etc., provided general care to patients during the course of examinations, inserted rectal tubes for barium enema examinations, prepared opaque media and equipment for examinations, cleaned syringes, catheters, etc., and made up trays and packages for subsequent sterilization.

They processed radiographs and ciné films in automatic processors and tanks or by Polaroid or other methods. They maintained and serviced automatic processing equipment.

They served on teams using mobile equipment in the Emergency Suite, the operating rooms and at the bedside. They became indispensable to the technologists in charge of these teams in moving equipment, positioning of patients and cassettes, in processing of radiographs, in running errands and in countless other ways.

They also assisted technologists with patients receiving therapeutic radiation or undergoing radioisotopic studies, particularly in transportation and patient watching. They assisted in the filing of radiographs and related clerical duties.

The major effort was in practical training; however, some

280 hours were devoted to didactic exercises conducted by instructors already serving in the school of radiologic technology. Particular emphasis was placed on radiation protection, management of patients during diagnostic procedures, nursing procedures involving detailed instruction in aseptic and antiseptic techniques, dark room chemistry and technique and office procedures and filing.

Twelve of the 15 students graduated and all proved employable, receiving salaries and other prerequisites in the range provided by the hospital for orderlies or ward secretaries.

A career ladder was built into the program whereby qualified aides might enter a school of radiologic technology, taking a high school equivalency examination (GED) if necessary, but none have done so to date.

In evaluating the students, throughout the program both written and practical tests were given at frequent intervals. The most important part of the evaluation was derived, however, from observation of students by their supervisors who met periodically to review the program and revise it as indicated. The reactions of the staff radiologic technologists, radiologists and residents were uniformly favorable and, in fact, enthusiastic.

LICENSURE

New York was the first state to establish a law requiring licensure for persons other than physicians and other licensed practitioners who are applying ionizing radiation to human beings, the Legislature enacting a bill as Chapter 295 of the Laws of 1964, effective on July 1, 1964.

The new law set forth conditions under which licensed persons could apply ionizing radiation. It also provided for examination and licensing of practicing technicians and set standards for training and licensing of future practitioners.

Prior to the enactment of the licensure bill, it had been estimated that there were 12,000–14,000 people who regularly exposed their fellow beings to radiation in New York State, only about 2,000 of whom had qualified as registrants of the ARRT.

During the first two years after the licensing bill went into effect, the State Health Department licensed about 6,800 individuals. It is assumed that most of the remainder eliminated themselves by not applying.

Under the new law, New York State, which had been notorious for the paucity of excellent training programs in radiologic technology, developed a number of new innovative programs, especially in community colleges, and upgraded existing programs. This pioneer legislation set high standards for eligibility for licensure for both existing and future practitioners of radiologic technology.

By 1972, California, New Jersey and Puerto Rico had also enacted licensure legislation of a comparable nature. A number of other states had similar bills introduced in their legislatures or on the planning boards.

UNIONIZATION

Unionization, which was long anathema to organized radiologic technology as well as to radiology, is now being given a hard second look by many thoughtful, conscientious radiologic technologists who find themselves locked into relatively low-paying jobs with little chance for advancement—all of this in an inflationary economy.

The rapidly advancing invasion of labor unions into hospital employment circles has recently been the subject of two well-documented and thoughtful studies made by the American College of Radiology and the journal, *Applied Radiology*.

On a regulatory level, the National Labor Relations Act applies to private hospitals but does not affect government or non-profit hospitals. There is, however, a bill before Congress (H.R. 11357) which, if enacted, would extend the Labor Act to non-profit hospitals. It is generally expected that this, or some similar bill, will pass and thus open the door to extensive inroads by unions.

The commonest issues are the economic ones: low wages, short vacations, lack of job security or seniority rights or adequate opportunity for advancement.

The June-July 1972 issue of *Applied Radiology* reported on

interviews of a dozen radiologists, radiologic technologists, and personnel directors of hospitals and clinics, and summarized their views of unionization as it affects hospital and clinic employment of health professionals.[40]

The AR survey found that most technologists recoil from strikes even when they support everything else unionization implies. Robert Best, Executive Director of ASRT stated, "Striking . . . isn't healthy for management or the allied health professional people and it isn't necessarily healthy for the patient either. We are not opposed to use of collective bargaining as a tool with which to improve economic status but. . . . The strike is still regarded as a non-professional technique and our members consider themselves professional."

THE FUTURE: WHAT DOES IT HOLD FOR RADIOLOGIC TECHNOLOGY?

Looking into the crystal ball involves predictable and unpredictable hazards.

Several of the manpower studies performed about ten years ago predicted, on what was then apparently sound evidence, that a distressing shortage of radiologists was already present and would become increasingly more pronounced even with full utilization of facilities for training residents. Due to a variety of factors, then not anticipated, it now seems that a shortage no longer exists or at least has become minimized.

The same may be true of radiologic technologists, particularly at the staff or lower echelon levels. Even in 1966, at the closing session of the National Conference on X-ray Technologist Training, Dr. Harold O. Peterson, then Chairman of the ACR Commission on Technologist Affairs asked "Is there truly a shortage?" It was his impression that shortages and overages were largely regional; that no real shortage existed in many metropolitan areas. However, loss of one or two technologists from a small hospital, especially in a rural area, creates a serious shortage in that community. Dr. Peterson ascribed shortages as due in part to the high attrition rate, particularly among females, and to the absence of many factors necessary to attract males into the field.

Since 1966 many new influences have been brought to bear in the manpower and womanpower field. Among these have been: 1) the leveling off of population growth from efforts on the part of young couples to limit the number of their off-spring, symbolized by "Zero Population Growth;" 2) the popu-larity of "Woman's Lib" with entrance of hordes of former housewives into careers in business and the professions; 3) the increasing inflationary rise in costs of life necessities; 4) in the field of radiology, the possibilities present for married female technologists to obtain employment—full-time, part-time or odd-time; 5) the truly remarkable growth in number of stu-dents trained in schools of radiologic technology.

All of these factors have undoubtedly contributed to al-leviating the shortages predicted ten years ago.

In 1962, there were 718 AMA approved schools with the capacity for training 7,739 students and 2,315 graduates, as shown in Table 1. A decade later, 1,113 schools comprising 1,554 clinical facilities had a total student capacity of 19,021 and listed 6,661 graduates.

Certainly, the most serious recent shortages in radiologic technology have been in the senior technologist areas, particu-larly in the categories of instructors and administrative per-sonnel, and in the subspecialty fields of special procedures, radiation therapy and nuclear medicine. It is hoped that the new programs, like those described above, will alleviate these shortages, especially if a career ladder can be implemented with opportunities for advancement, both professionally and financially (Table 2).

Our experience with Radiology Aides has convinced us that these low echelon workers have proven a most welcome and competent addition to a busy radiology department and have been able to relieve the more highly trained technologist from many chores.

As the impact of the development of degree-offering prog-rams begins to be felt about the country, it seems apparent that a number of certificate hospital-based programs will be gradually phased out. However, the new program at Duke encourages the continuation of hospital-based schools in North Carolina, with Duke providing educational facilities

Table 2

A Career Ladder Concept in Radiologic Technology

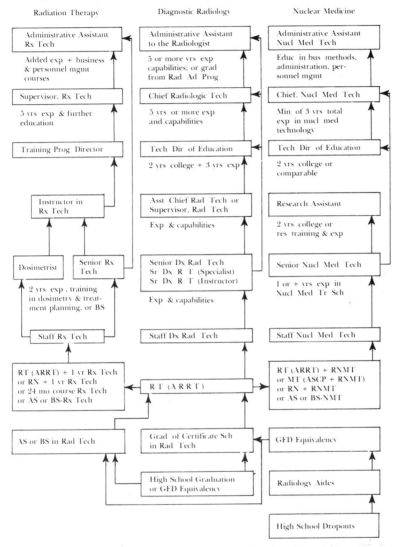

Other Professionals: radiologists, clinical or academic; other MD specialists in nuclear medicine; radiological physicists; radiobiologists; radiochemists; radiological engineers; radiological health specialists; radiation safety officers; radiological physics technologists; radiological health technologists.

Other Supporting Personnel: radiologic librarians; secretarial, clerical and filing personnel; computer specialists; radiological group or dept. business mgr.; machine service personnel; operators of semi-automated radiographic equipment; dark room workers; loaders of automated film viewers; mould technicians.

which permit qualified graduates of certificate schools to continue on to educational programs designed to produce
teachers, administrators and other specialists.

George F. Koenig, past president of the ASRT, speaking
before the Association of University Radiologic Technologists
in 1970,[41] noted that most radiologic technologists were still
produced by on-the-job training in some 1,300 hospital-based
schools which lack educators and suitable facilities and are not
equipping technologists to function adequately in the modern, sophisticated environment of hospital radiology departments. He felt that technology should be taught at a much
higher level and recommended that the junior college programs should replace the non-degree hospital-based schools
and that baccalaureate programs should be expanded and
enriched in order to prepare qualified students for careers in
administrative and teaching positions, as radiologists' assistants and in other subspecialties.

One reservation regarding the phasing out of the hospital-
based schools is that they have provided vocational training
for a number of young people whose parents were economically disadvantaged and could not afford to send their children to college.

Many of the community college programs, especially those
supported by state appropriations, have been able to maintain
relatively low tuition levels, but this is not universal.

At the University of Vermont, for example, an educationally sound two-year certificate program with 70 students enrolled at the Medical Center Hospital of Vermont cost the
students virtually nothing except for books and uniforms.

As this program was phased out to be replaced by an
associate's degree program at the university, students in the
new school were required to pay an annual tuition of $950 if
they lived in the New England States or of $2,400 if they were
from out-of-area. Room and meals averaged $1,000 a year;
books, uniforms and fees added another $271.50. While some
aid is available in the form of scholarships and low interest
loans, a number of students have to go deeply in debt before
they graduate and complete their requirements for registration.

In areas where college costs are relatively high, it seems apparent that a large pool of qualified but impecunious young men and women is being lost to the field.

Equivalency and Proficiency Testing. It seems probable that equivalency and proficiency examinations may be developed soon in order to permit qualified students to receive credit for knowledge already attained in applying for admission to degree programs with advanced class standing. Some colleges and universities are allowing two to four semesters of credit for training received in certain certificate schools. However, such is still not possible in many four-year institutions.

Equivalency examinations would open doors to many experienced and intelligent technologists who are now held back by the conventional stringent requirements for admission to most baccalaureate programs.

That occupational proficiency examinations for radiologic technologists may become a reality is suggested by the recent award of a contract to Educational Testing Services, Princeton, New Jersey, by the National Institutes of Health for development of such examinations.[42]

If successful, a mechanism might be established to provide access to credentials for persons trained in nonacademic environments, thus contributing significantly to the rate of a technologist's progression toward a position with increased responsibility and commensurate salary.

Future Trends in the Education of Radiologic Technologists. In a carefully researched and thoughtfully written three-part article, *Radiologic Technology Education: an Overview*, Carol Schmidt, one of the Feature Editors of the new journal, *Applied Radiology*, presents a comprehensive and penetrating survey of the field,[43] based on interviews of a dozen leading figures in the areas of education and accreditation of technologists.

Their views were divergent, as might be expected. Most agreed, however, that significant strides had been made in the past decade in the development of more and better educational opportunities in both the certificate and degree schools.

The article does not lend itself to condensation and should be read in its entirety by those interested in present and future trends in the education and certification of technologists at all levels.

It did seem apparent to some of those interviewed (and to this observer) that many of the hospital-based programs must be relied upon for years to come in order to produce an adequate supply of technologists for employment at the staff level. It is hoped that these programs will be upgraded by employment of graduates of degree schools as teachers and supervisors. It is also a fact that many graduates of certificate programs have no desire or perhaps ability to progress beyond the level for which they are trained.

Limited Service Workers. With the development of automated and semi-automated equipment, there will undoubtedly be pressures to utilize personnel who have been trained to perform one task only—comparable to the operators of photo-roentgen chest units of past years.

Some licensure laws prevent persons with limited skills from operating such equipment but there are several possible solutions: 1) to examine and license operators for performance of limited tasks, as is permissible in California; 2) to utilize non-licensed radiology aides who would be trained to set up patients under the general supervision of a licensed radiologic technologist who would make the actual exposures. It has been suggested that a department could be planned so that one registered technologist could control perhaps half a dozen machines, on each of which a patient would be set up by the aides; the technologist would then check the positioning, tube placement, etc., and then make the radiographic exposure.

LICENSURE

The omens portend to this amateur soothsayer that licensure of persons applying ionizing radiation to humans and certification of educational facilities concerned with training of such workers will soon be the law of the land in all fifty states.

Since radiation received from the medical and dental use of x-ray and from radionuclides is by far the largest source of ionizing radiation received by human beings, it is only rational to believe that the public will demand that this be administered only by persons of proven capability.

It is to be hoped that there will be sufficient uniformity in state licensure and certification laws to provide reciprocal arrangements which would permit license-holders from one state to move to another with a minimum of expense and red tape as job opportunities occur. Ideally, licensure and certification should be based on national standards. If the legislation now in Congress is enacted, this will assure relative uniformity in the licensure laws of the various states.

UNIONIZATION

The rapid spread of unionization in states which permit it and the likelihood of passage of H.R. 11357 which would, in effect, provide that non-profit hospitals be declared suitable for collective bargaining, will undoubtedly stimulate the organization of hospital employees at an unprecedented rate. Unions will probably be successful in being designated as the bargaining groups in many institutions. However, if organized radiology and organized radiologic technology have their way, collective bargaining will be conducted by national or local technologist societies; if this comes about, strikes, which are abhorrent to most technologists, will be virtually barred.

EPILOGUE

Radiologic technology has completed more than fifty years of existence and has developed into one of the major allied health professions. From small beginnings in the early 1920s, it has survived many crises and has surmounted innumerable problems in developing satisfactory educational programs and creating adequate opportunities for career advancement.

While other stormy days undoubtedly lie ahead, its future seems well assured—largely because of the continuing influ-

ence of an outstanding group of leaders in the field, dedicated
to the development of educational programs of a high degree
of excellence and the maintenance of professionalism in their
relationships with the institutions in which they serve.

NOTES

1. Otto Glasser, *Wilhelm Conrad Röntgen and the Early History of the Roentgen Rays* (Springfield, Ill.: Charles C. Thomas, 1934); Ruth and Edward Brecher, *The Rays; a History of Radiology in the United States and Canada* (Baltimore: Williams and Wilkins Co., 1969).

2. Percy Brown, *American Martyrs to Science through the Roentgen Rays* (Springfield, Ill.: Charles C. Thomas, 1936).

3. E. A. Codman, *Philadelphia Medical Journal* 9 (1902):438.

4. Paul C. Hodges, "A Radiological Odyssey," *The Pharos* 36 (1973):2.

5. Ed. C. Jerman, *Modern X-ray Technic* (St. Paul-Minneapolis, Minn.: Bruce Publishing Co., 1928).

6. The American Registry of Radiologic Technologists, 2600 Wayzata Boulevard, Minneapolis, Minnesota 55455.

7. The American Society of Radiologic Technologists, 645 North Michigan Avenue, Suite 620, Chicago, Illinois 60611.

8. Alfred B. Greene, "Quo Fata Vocant," *The X-ray Technician* 26 (1954):76.

9. The American College of Radiology, 20 North Wacker Drive, Chicago, Illinois 60606.

10. Department of Allied Medical Professions and Services, Division of Medical Education, American Medical Association, 535 North Dearborn Street, Chicago, Illinois 60610.

11. *Curriculum and Teacher's Syllabus for Schools of X-ray Technology; a Teaching Guide,* American Society of Radiologic Technologists, Chicago, Illinois (1966).

12. *Allied Health Education Programs in Junior Colleges/1970,* compiled by American Association of Junior Colleges, Department of Health, Education and Welfare Publication No. (NIH) 72-163.

13. National Advisory Committee on Radiation, "Protecting and Improving Health Through the Radiological Sciences: A Surgeon General Report." National Center for Radiologic Health, Public Health Service, Rockville, Md., 1966.

14. *Report of the Medical X-ray Advisory Committee on Public Health*. "Considerations in Medical Diagnostic Radiology (X-rays)," USPHS, Washington, D.C., 1967.

15. *Report of the Commission on Cost of Medical Care*, Vol. I, American Medical Association, Chicago, Illinois, 1964.

16. United States Department of Labor: Health Manpower 1966-75: "A Study of Requirements and Supply," *Bureau of Labor Statistics Report* 323, Washington, D.C., 1967; United States Department of Labor: Technology and Manpower in the Health Service Industry, 1965-1975. Manpower Research Bull. No. 14, Washington, D.C., 1967; USPHS: "Education for the Allied Health Professions and Services," *Report of the Allied Health Professions Education Subcommittee of the National Advisory Health Council*. PHS Publication 1600, Bureau of Health Manpower, Washington, D.C., 1967.

17. Roland C. McGowan, Executive Director, American Registry of Radiologic Technologists, Minneapolis, Minn. Personal Communication, Dec. 1967.

18. National Conference on X-ray Technician Training, Center of Adult Education, University of Maryland, College Park, Md., Sept. 7-9, 1966. *Proceedings*. National Center for Radiologic Health, PHS, Rockville, Md., 1967.

19. Mary Ellen Hughes, R.T. (ARRT), Secretary, Joint Review Committee on Education in Radiologic Technology. Personal Communication, Feb. 9, 1973; Warren G. Ball, D.D.S., Assistant Director, Department of Allied Medical Professions and Services, Division of Medical Education, American Medical Association, Chicago, Illinois. Personal Communication, March 2, 1973.

20. Joint Review Committee on Education in Radiologic Technology, 307 North Michigan Avenue, Suite 1801, Chicago, Illinois 60601.

21. *Essentials of an Accredited Educational Program for Radiologic Technologists*, Revised December, 1969; Council on Medical Education, American Medical Association, 535 North Dearborn Street, Chicago, Illinois 60610.

22. *Essentials of an Acceptable School of Radiation Therapy Technology*, AMA Council on Medical Education with the cooperation of the ACR, ARRT, and the ASRT; Approved Dec. 1, 1968 by the House of Delegates of the AMA.

23. *Essentials of an Approved Educational Program for Radiation Therapy Technologists–Two-year Program*, Revised December 1972; Established by AMA Council on Medical Education in collaboration with American College of Radiology; American Society of Radiologic Technologists.

24. *Essentials of an Accredited Educational Program in Nuclear Medicine Technology*, AMA Council on Medical Education in collaboration with the ACR, ASCP, ASMT, ASRT and SNMT; Approved July 1969 by AMA House of Delegates. *Radiologic Technology* 41 (1969):139.

25. *Study of Accreditation of Selected Health Educational Programs*, Commission Report. National Commission on Accrediting, 1972. SASHEP, Suite 760, One Dupont Circle, N.W., Washington, D.C. 20036.

26. Guy H. Simmons, J. G. Kereiakes, and H. N. Welman, "Educational Program in Nuclear Medicine Technology," *JAMA* 217, No. 8 (1971):1082; James G. Kereiakes, *et al.*, "Degree Associated Training Programs in Nuclear Medicine Technology," *Practical Radiology* 1, No. 3 (1973):40.

27. *Development of Career Opportunities for Nuclear Medicine Technologists: A Report on the Application of the Career Ladder Concept to the Field of Nuclear Medicine Technology; May 1972*. Technical Education Research Center, Cambridge, Mass. 02138.

28. *Nuclear Medical Technology Training:* Proceedings of a Colloquium held on Feb. 28, 1969, at the Radioisotope Laboratory, Cincinnati General Hospital, Cincinnati, Ohio; June 1971, Bureau of Radiological Health, PHS, FDA, U.S. Dept. HEW. Rockville, Md. 20852. (FDA) 72-8002, 1971.

29. Benjamin Felson, *et al.*, "The Radiology Administrator," *Radiology* 97 (1970):191; W. J. Bunnell, *et al.*, "Radiologic Administration: A Professional Niche for Technology," *Radiologic Technology* 43 (1971):24.

30. *The Training of Radiologic Administrators:* Proceedings of a Symposium held in Cincinnati, Ohio, May 22, 1970. Bureau of Rad. Health, PHS, FDA, U.S. Dept. of HEW; DHEW Pub. No. (FDA) 72-8023.

31. J. A. Campbell, *et al.*, "Experience with Technician Performance of Gastrointestinal Examinations," *Radiology* 92 (1969):65; W. J. Tuddenham, *et al.*, "Preliminary Evaluation of Effectiveness of Logical Flow Charts in Teaching Roentgen Diagnosis," *Radiology* 93 (1969):17; F. S. Alcorn, *et al.*, "The Protocol and Results of Training Non-radiologists to Scan Mammograms," *Radiology* 99 (1971):523; and D. J. Sheft, *et al.*, "Screening of Chest Roentgenograms by Advanced Roentgen Technologists," *Radiology* 94 (1970):427.

32. Edward J. Huber, "A Program to Train Physicians' Assistants in Diagnostic Radiology," *Applied Radiology* 3 (1974):31.

33. Thomas T. Thompson, *et al.*, "New Opportunities for Radiologic Technologists: Physician's Assistant in Radiology," *Radiologic Technology* 42 (1970):8.

34. Thomas T. Thompson, *et al.*, *The Subjective Evaluation of Physician's Assistants in Radiology; The Objective Evaluation of Physician's Assistants in Radiology.* Duke University Medical Center and VA Hospital, Durham, N.C.

35. John B. Cahoon, R.T., F.A.S.R.T., Assistant Professor and Director,

Radiologic Technology Programs. Duke University Medical Center, Durham, N.C. Personal Communication, Feb. 21, 1973.

36. William R. Hendee, "Changing Patterns in the Training of Radiologic Technologists; A Case Report," *Radiologic Technology* 42 (1971):392.

37. See notes number 13 and 14 above.

38. A. Bradley Soule, "Radiology Aides: An Editorial," *Radiology* 104 (1972):215.

39. *Manpower Development and Training Act of 1962*, as Amended, Aug. 1968. Public Law 90-490S.

40. Marilyn Farley, "When Technologists Join Unions," *Applied Radiology* 1 (June-July 1972):23.

41. George F. Koenig, "Restructuring the Education of Radiologic Technologists," *Radiologic Technology* 43 (1971):127.

42. William R. Hendee, "Proficiency and Equivalency in Radiologic Technology: Guest Editorial," *Applied Radiology* 1, No. 4 (1972):10.

43. Carol Schmidt, "Radiologic Technology Education: An Overview," *Applied Radiology* 1, No. 4 (1972):53; 2, No. 1 (1973):45; 2, No. 2 (1973).

EVOLUTION OF THE PHYSICIAN'S ASSISTANT

D. Robert Howard & David E. Lewis

The disparity between the demand for and availability of primary health care services has continued to grow in the past decade. Efforts to remedy this problem have included increasing the number of trained physicians, the utilization of computer technology and the development of new roles for physician's assistants, nurses, and other health workers so that a greater share of the physician's burden can be borne by non-physicians. The latter, though still in the experimental phase, have clearly demonstrated their potential worth.

The discussion of physician's assistants here will relate to the Type A category as defined by the National Academy of Sciences in 1970. By its definition, this type of physician's assistant "is capable of approaching the patient, collecting historical and physical data, organizing the data, and presenting them in such a way that the physician can visualize the medical problem and determine appropriate diagnostic or therapeutic steps. He is also capable of assisting the physician by performing diagnostic and therapeutic procedures and coordinating the roles of other more technical assistants. While he functions under the general supervision and responsibility of the physician, he might under special circumstances and under defined rules, perform without the immediate surveillance of the physician. He is, thus, distinguished by his ability to integrate and interpret findings on the basis of general medical knowledge to exercise a degree of independent judgment."[1]

The Background

Program Development. Duke University initiated the first formalized program for the training of physician's assistants in 1965. Dr. Eugene A. Stead, Jr., then Chairman of the Department of Medicine at Duke, recognized the plight of the overworked primary care practitioners and saw the potential of providing former military corpsmen with further medical training that would enable them to effectively and safely augment the physicians' service capability. He felt that corpsmen, with additional medical training, could function at a professional level and—under the direction and supervision of a physician—carry out many functions traditionally performed exclusively by physicians, thereby extending the physician's reach to a greater patient population. Since 1965, a formalized two-year program consisting of nine months of basic science preparation augmented with 15 months of clinical training, has evolved at Duke University.

At the same time, a similar effort to train physician's assistants was instituted at the University of Kentucky by the joint efforts of Dr. Joseph Hamburg, the Dean of the College of Allied Health Professions at the University of Kentucky Medical Center, and Dr. Robert Ewer, a practicing internist in Evansville, Indiana.

By the end of 1969, physician's assistant programs were operating at the Federal Bureau of Prisons in Springfield, Missouri; Bowman Gray School of Medicine at Winston-Salem, North Carolina; and Alderson-Broaddus College at Philippi, West Virginia.

Funding Resources. Funding for physician's assistant programs came exclusively from private, non-governmental sources until 1971, when the United States Congress passed the Comprehensive Health Manpower Act that provided support for physician's assistant training through the Office of Special Programs. It was stated at that time that the Bureau of Health Manpower Education would continue this project on an annual basis for a period of three to five years, dependent upon the demonstrated success of the concept, the av-

ailability of appropriations, a demonstrated need, and satisfactory performance by the contractors. In 1972, thirty-nine
programs were funded by the Office of Special Programs,
Bureau of Health Manpower Education, Department of
Health, Education and Welfare.[2]

The MEDEX Concept. The MEDEX concept, which began in
June of 1969 at the University of Washington, was a parallel
effort to produce physician's assistants that also consisted of a
mix of didactic and clinical teaching but placed primary emphasis on the performance of tasks. The first MEDEX program, at the University of Washington, was funded by the
National Center for Health Services Research and Development of the Health Services and Mental Health Administration, within the Department of Health, Education and
Welfare.

As a result of the early acceptance of the MEDEX concept,
eight similar programs were also slated for funding and
implementation. One of the settings, the University of
Alabama, was unique in that it instituted both a Duke-type
physician's assistant program and a MEDEX program. The
latter has since been discontinued.

*Factors Influencing the Growth of Physician's Assistant
Programs.* Because current social, economic and political factors preclude the possibility of educating physicians in sufficient numbers to be the sole providers of high quality,
comprehensive health care services, the only way physicians
can meet their professional responsibilities efficiently and
effectively is by rational task delegation to non-physicians who
are trained to be competent in performing specific functions
directly related to patient care.

The need for additional health professionals has evolved
because of two major changes in the health care industry:
first, the shift in emphasis from purely medical care to total
and comprehensive health care and, second, the ability of
more and more people to afford health and medical services.
The ability to pay for medical care, which is a result of the
increased availability of health insurance, personal economic

gains or various federally sponsored insurance programs, will likely be of increasing importance in the future.

One other factor that influenced the evolution of programs to train physician's assistants during the early years was the relative scarcity of nursing personnel and the availability of ex-military corpsmen. Approximately 20,000 of the then 60,000 men discharged from the armed forces each year with two to three years of medical training wanted a career in the civilian health care services industry. Physician's assistant programs were initially developed primarily to make use of this manpower resource. However, the Army, Navy and Air Force are now operating programs of their own to train physician's assistants, draining off much of this once abundant source.

Because of the resulting scarcity of candidates for civilian training programs, applicants with backgrounds in most health related fields are now being considered. This has, in turn, generated an even greater manpower pool from which to draw.

A report of the Association of American Medical Colleges, entitled *Media Utilization and Needs in Physician's Assistant Programs and Related Medical-Health Education*, was clearly one of the most significant undertakings in 1972 relating to the physician's assistant concept.

The specific purpose of the study was to determine the types of media and multi-media hardware currently being used for instruction in physician's assistant programs and to identify the priority needs of the programs for new media and/or multi-media materials. While the report concentrates mainly on physician's assistant programs, the investigators also examined the application of the same media materials to other areas of medical-health education, including nursing, other allied health occupations and undergraduate, graduate and postgraduate physician education.

This study is intended to be the first of a three-phase project. It will be augmented by a second phase that will involve the design, production and testing of a pilot media system in the primary area of identified need which will embody the highest possible quality in content and integrated methods of presentation. The third phase, by utilizing the concept of cooperative design and execution, will involve the development of similar multi-media units covering other priority subjects identified in the listing of determined needs.

Data from this report revealed that the professionally-related training for physician's assistants ranges from 12 to 24 months in length. So far as the division of this time into didactic and clinical components is concerned, anywhere from 20 to 50 percent of the time is spent in didactic teaching with the average being less than 40 percent.

The annual enrollment in 1972 of the 22 programs investigated was reported to be 713, with a projected enrollment in the next five years of 880.

A comparison of the prerequisites for admission and student profiles showed that most students actually have more education and experience than the minimum prerequisites.[3]

"THE PHYSICIAN'S ASSISTANT— TODAY AND TOMORROW"

A book published in 1972 is, without doubt, the single most comprehensive source of information available to date on the physician's assistant concept.[4] The book is *The Physician's Assistant–Today and Tomorrow*, by Alfred M. Sadler, Jr., M.D.; Blair L. Sadler, J.D., and Ann A. Bliss, R.N., M.S.W.

William Stanhope, Director of the Oklahoma Physician's Associate Program, in a review of the book stated "the authors have summarized, in an exemplary manner, the concepts, concerns and legal issues central to the implementation and conceptual utilization of the Physician's Assistant," and "the authors deserve to be especially commended for the concluding chapter which very astutely reviews the major issues confronting Physician's Assistants and the concept as a whole."[5]

PERTINENT LEGISLATION

In the spring of 1968 a conference was held to investigate the legal status of physician's assistants. It was attended by leaders of the North Carolina State Medical Society (including representatives of the Legislative Committee and Medico-legal Committee), the North Carolina Board of Medical Examiners, the North Carolina Nurses' Association, the American Medical Association and individuals from schools planning the development of such programs.[6]

A supplemental legal conference was held in October, 1969, to determine the most desirable and feasible means of accommodating emerging groups of allied health professionals into the legal framework of medical practice. This conference was sponsored by the federal Department of Health, Education and Welfare (HEW) in conjunction with the Department of Community Health Sciences at Duke University. At that conference five alternative courses of action were presented for consideration: 1) maintaining the status quo (i.e., doing nothing); 2) licensing physician's assistants; 3) enacting a general statute authorizing supervised delegations by physicians; 4) special licensing of physicians to utilize physician's assistants; and 5) establishing a Committee on Health Manpower Innovations to control the development and utilization of new personnel.

The ultimate consensus was that efforts should be directed initially toward the drafting of a general statute authorizing supervised delegations by physicians, with the responsibility for determining which persons may accept such delegations vested in the State Board of Medical Examiners.[7]

John Ball, J.D., legal consultant to the Duke University Physician's Associate Program and director of the legislative development project, reported at the annual conference of New Health Practitioners in New Orleans that as of April, 1974, 32 states had enacted some type of legislation relating to physician's assistants.

National Conferences

As the first institution to establish a formal program for educating and training physician's assistants, Duke University sponsored a series of conferences covering various aspects of the physician's assistant concept in order to share its experiences and learn from the experiences of others.[8]

The Fourth Annual Conference, held in April of 1972, dealt with numerous issues of current importance relating to the physician's assistant concept. Included were review of the status of current legislation, educational essentials, and the function and utilization of nurses functioning in an expanded role; workshops dealt with the use of physician's assistants in primary care, the use of physician's assistants in referral care, and the curricular and administrative problems experienced by six physician's assistant programs from across the country.[9]

During the 1972 Conference, the administrators of the Duke Physician's Associate Program recommended—because of the great proliferation of programs designed to train "assistants to the primary care physician"—that the sponsorship of the annual national conferences be rotated.

THE ASSOCIATION OF PHYSICIAN ASSISTANT PROGRAMS

In 1970 the American Registry of Physician's Associates was formed by representatives of established programs to provide a mechanism for registering and recognizing graduates of quality programs and others who, through non-traditional and informal training, were capable of performing in an equally competent manner. The functions and roles of the Registry were limited, however, in that its membership was comprised exclusively of representatives of two-year physician's assistant programs. One other purpose of this organization was to stimulate interest by organized medicine to participate in the development of national certification procedures.

By 1972 the membership of the American Registry of Physician's Associates recognized that their original goals were being achieved. It was also realized that there was a need for cooperative development of the educational processes among the many programs training physician's assistants. Accordingly, at a meeting held in Atlanta, the membership of the Registry voted to form a new organization entitled "The Association of Physician Assistant Programs." The primary purposes of this new organization were to create a forum for physician's assistant program personnel and to serve as the spokesman for physician's assistant programs. As of April, 1974, the Association of Physician Assistant Programs had a membership of 45.[10]

The objectives of the APAP are:

1) Assist in the development and organization of educational curricula for physician assistant programs so as to better assure the public of competent physician assistants.

2) Assist in the defining of the roles of physician assistants in the field of medicine so as to maximize the benefit to the public of their services.

3) Establish and/or encourage the establishment of continuing educational programs for physician assistants so as to assure the public the benefits of new medical discoveries and improved medical techniques.

4) Coordinate program logistics such as admissions and career placements in an effort to meet the public's growing and continuing need for medical services,

5) Continuously evaluate the programs so as to assure the public of properly trained physician assistants,

6) Serve as a public information center with respect to its programs.

THE ROLE OF ORGANIZED MEDICINE

In November, 1968, the American Medical Association's Council on Medical Education was approached regarding the establishment of educational essentials. In accordance with guidelines put into effect at that time, the matter was transferred to the Council on Health Manpower for study and recommendations. During the years 1969 and 1970 the Council on Health Manpower drafted *Guidelines for Development of New Health Occupations*, which were adopted by the American Medical Association's House of Delegates in 1970.

Within the directives of these Guidelines, a task force comprised of representatives from the American Society of Internal Medicine, the American College of Physicians, and the American Academy of Family Physicians drafted a document defining the need for, role and functions of the primary physician's assistant. This document was submitted to the Council on Health Manpower which approved the proposal on April 17, 1971. By the end of April the Advisory Committee on Education for the Allied Health Professions and Services of the American Medical Association's Council on Medical Education received this information and established a subcommittee to draft educational essentials.

The subcommittee, comprised of representatives from the AMA, the sponsoring specialty organizations, the Association of American Medical Colleges, the American Academy of Pediatrics, and five physician's assistant programs met in May and again in August of 1971. By the conclusion of the second meeting a draft for the *Essentials of an Approved Educational Program for the Assistant to the Primary Care Physician* was unanimously adopted. (In order to bypass the very involved nomenclature issues, the subcommittee agreed to generically classify this new health professional as "the assistant to the primary care physician.")

Between September and November, 1971, the *Essentials* were approved by four of the sponsoring specialty organizations. (The Association of American Medical Colleges withdrew as a sponsoring organization because of a differing view as to the appropriate methodology for implementing approval.) Following final approval by the Council on Medical Education, the *Essentials* were officially enacted by a vote of the American Medical Association's House of Delegates on November 30, 1971.

The *Essentials* describe the assistant to the primary care physician as "a skilled person, qualified by academic and clinical training to provide patient services under the supervision and responsibility of a doctor of medicine or osteopathy who is, in turn, responsible for the performance of that assistant. The assistant may be involved with the patients of the physician in any medical setting for which the physician is responsible."[11]

To be accredited by the AMA, a program must have a formal curriculum that prepares its graduates to provide the following eight types of patient services:

1) The initial approach to a patient of any age group in any

setting to elicit a detailed and accurate history, perform an appropriate physical examination, and record and present pertinent data in a manner meaningful to the physician;

2) Performance and/or assistance in performance of routine laboratory and related studies as appropriate for a specific practice setting, such as the drawing of blood samples, performance of urinalyses, and the taking of electrocardiographic tracings;

3) Performance of such routine therapeutic procedures as injections, immunizations, and the suturing and care of wounds;

4) Instruction and counseling of patients regarding physical and mental health on matters such as diets, disease, therapy, and normal growth and development;

5) Assisting the physician in the hospital setting by making patient rounds, recording patient progress notes, accurately and appropriately transcribing and/or executing standing orders and other specific orders at the direction of the supervising physician, and compiling and recording detailed narrative case summaries;

6) Providing assistance in the delivery of service to patients requiring continuing care (home, nursing home, extended care faciliites, etc.), including the review and monitoring of treatment and therapy plans;

7) Independent performance of evaluative and treatment procedures essential to provide an appropriate response to life-threatening, emergency situations; and

8) Facilitation of the physician's referral of appropriate patients by maintenance of an awareness of the community's various health facilities, agencies, and resources.

As of April, 1974, 43 programs had received approval from the American Medical Association.

NATIONAL CERTIFICATION PROGRAM

In 1972, the National Board of Medical Examiners, with the concurrence and cooperation of the AMA's Council on Health Manpower, embarked upon a national program to certify assistants to the primary care physician.[12]

This new role for the National Board emerged after extensive study and discussion that continued over many months. The question was considered in depth by the Board's Committee on Goals and Priorities, which undertook a review of the most likely course for medical education and the related needs of evaluation and certification over the next ten years. A report prepared by two members of this Committee, Miss Margaret E. Mahoney, Vice-President, The Robert Wood Johnson Foundation, and Dr. John E. Evans, President, The University of Toronto, dealt in a very compelling manner with the rapidly moving events that led to the recommendation that the National Board assume responsibility for developing examinations for physician's assistants.

A Special Study Committee under the chairmanship of Edmund D. Pellegrino, M.D., Vice-President for Health Sciences, State University of New York at Stonybrook, was appointed.

In order to identify the specific competencies of the physician's assistant, a task inventory consisting of some nine hundred health care tasks was compiled. These tasks were organized under five major headings which represented various components of the clinical problem-solving process: data gathering, data analysis and interpretation, data synthesis, medical and health care procedures, and other health care activities. Each of these major headings was then divided into subcategories in which tasks of a similar nature were grouped.

Because the number of health care tasks that the physician's assistant should be able to perform is so large, it became evident that it would not be possible to sample each of these tasks adequately on a certifying examination. For this reason, the Committee was asked to establish priorities for these tasks on the basis of how frequently they would be encountered in the practice of a primary care physician, and how critical they are to optimum health care delivery. Therefore, in a second inventory, the Committee members were asked to evaluate each health care task on two scales, each consisting of four intervals indicating high-to-low frequency and high-to-low criticalness.

By March, 1973, the high priority health care task list was

completed. An analysis of the priority list served as the basis for formal evaluation materials, and a pilot test of various techniques took place in December, 1973.

A total of 882 students sat for the first exam; 62 percent were physician's assistants, 29 percent were MEDEX graduates and 9 percent were nurse practitioners.

CONCLUSION AND OPINIONS

National Leadership. A great weakness in the evolution of physician's assistants has been the almost total lack of any national, organized leadership to evaluate and monitor their development. There is a need now to implement a nationally coordinated series of evaluative studies relating to various aspects of physician's assistants roles.

First, it is imperative that a study of the work/performance roles of various types of specialized and generalized physician's assistants be conducted to determine what specific functions physician's assistants are performing; how these vary within each subcategory; how they relate to patient care, administration, research and education; and the economic productivity of physician's assistants functioning in various occupational roles. A second survey that is sorely needed at this time is a comparative study of the educational processes and how they relate to the specific functions physician's assistants actually perform after graduation. This should be an ongoing effort so that the educational preparation of physician's assistants can be continually modified to fit them for the ever-changing role they will be assuming as members of the health team. Such an effort might preclude the type of stifling and inappropriate curricula that confront most other health occupational groups.

A comparative evaluation of the performance of physician's assistants as opposed to registered nurses functioning in expanded roles would also be valuable. It might reveal that the curricula of the two groups could be extensively coordinated.

With the findings of these studies, much-needed guidelines could be developed leading to optimal utilization patterns for physician's assistants. If liability is to be effectively limited in the future it is vitally important that skill and training of physician's assistants not only be put to optimum use but that specific guidelines be developed for employing and/or super-, vising physicians to follow in monitoring and evaluating their role in the health team. Such data would also enable physicians to define more accurately the precise makeup of a staff which could most effectively meet the specific needs of their individual practice.

Recent progress in developing a system of national certification for physician's assistants is probably the best example of how an issue pertaining to physician's assistants ought to be approached. The progress made under the leadership of the National Board of Medical Examiners during 1972 and 1973 was exemplary. Clearly the availability of a national means of classifying and certifying the competence of individual physician's assistants will be paramount in the development of this profession. If the certification procedure that evolves truly measures an individual's competence to perform in his anticipated role, it will not only serve to legitimize and stabilize the physician's assistant concept as a recognized profession but also act as a model for other health occupations.

One other area of need that will require national coordination is the creation of a single center for the placement of physician's assistants. There is little likelihood that a national employment center will effectively influence physician's assistants to settle in the places of greatest need, but it could provide them with the best opportunity to identify a practice setting that can most effectively meet their individual needs. A professional placement system, similar to the physician's placement service sponsored by the AMA, would be beneficial to both the physician's assistants and their potential employers.

Funding. One of the most serious problems that physician's assistant programs are likely to confront in the next few years is related to the tenuous status of funding sources. Virtually all of the early funding sources for physician's assistant programs are now practically defunct. Private sources, relied upon initially by many of the programs, contributed support primarily as seed money to see this innovative concept through its early experimental phases. The MEDEX programs, which received initial funding from the Health Services and Mental Health Administration, now also must seek continued support from other sources.

Current funding, available through the federal government via the Office of Special Projects in the Bureau of Health Manpower Education, is totally insufficient to provide any realistic degree of support for meeting the high costs of these educational programs. As has been the case in other health careers, it is unlikely that the federal government can be relied upon for any significant long-term support.

It seems fair to presume at this time that, if the federal government were to withdraw its financial support for physician's assistant programs, the majority of the programs would fold within a year or two. This is not to imply that the programs are unworthy, however, as discontinuation of federal support would put other health career training programs in jeopardy, as well.

The problems that will confront physician's assistant programs in the next decade will likely be shared by all health-related training programs. In all probability, most programs will have to look increasingly toward state and local governments for continued financial support. Many institutions also may find it necessary to reassess their priorities for the utilization of available funding and restructure their educational programs accordingly.

The present limitations in private, federal and state funding resources are likely to cause an increased reliance on patient fees for educational support. Such a return of the pendulum, however, is not wholly unwarranted in light of the facts that patient fees derived from institutional care are largely covered by insurance, and most people are presently covered by either private or federally sponsored insurance programs. The distribution of the burden in this manner might well be more equitable than one supported by taxes.

While future funding for physician's assistant programs will certainly create a severe problem, it is unlikely that the relative effect on physician's assistant programs will be disproportionate to that experienced by health training programs in general.

Planning. Perhaps the most difficult problem to be faced in the next decade will be related to planning based on anticipated future needs. In the past, the forecasts of many reliable organizations and individuals have varied widely and been similar only in their near-perfect record of inaccuracy. On the basis of the difficulty experienced by forecasters in the past, it is clear that one of the key issues of success will be in maintaining a significant degree of flexibility. This can be assured only by emphasizing educational concepts and developing problem solving skills.

While increased numbers of physician's assistants can be readily incorporated into the health care delivery system in this country, overproduction must be guarded against as this would create a condition equally unfair to both the provider and the consumer. Whatever planning for the future takes place must be multilateral and unemotional for—while physician's assistants are not the sole solution to the problems confronting the health services industry in this country—the possibility for any solution is unlikely without reliance on them to some degree. Keeping these two diverse factors in balance is essential to successful planning for the future.

The unpredictability of socially related influences will continue to be a primary problem in forecasting health manpower needs. In spite of the plethora of unknown factors, however, certain characteristics vital to the evolution of the physician's assistant must be considered as they relate to the future. First, because of the reduction in the size of the armed forces and the major commitment the military has made to the education and utilization of physician's assistants, ex-corpsmen with an interest in pursuing a career in the health field will be virtually non-existent in the future. This factor alone will precipitate major changes in the basic concept of physician's assistant training. People involved in the selection and training of physician's assistants will have to look to new sources of manpower. Clearly, one of the options will be to enroll high school graduates with no experience. Because of the maturity and judgement an individual must have to perform as a physician's assistant, programs designed for these students must be markedly expanded to include a major component of general education at the undergraduate college level.

A second alternative will be to select college graduates with no experience in the health field and provide them with a relatively comprehensive health-related education. If either of these options is to be selected, it will be necessary to more precisely investigate the relationship between "previous experience in a health-related career" and both the ability to perform as a physician's assistant as well as the effect of previous experience on career longevity.

A third option will be to select students from the ranks of the established health careers. This action might well result in the evolution of the physician's assistant role as one of vertical mobility in the health careers. Reliance on people with a background in a health occuption would necessarily include a significant number of nurses, and thereby might result in the nurse functioning in an expanded role.

Obviously, many arguments can be made in favor of or in opposition to any of these possibilities. However, if the physician's assistant profession is to move vertically on the health career ladder, many restrictive changes in the organization of existing health occupations will have to be overcome.

Another very definite trend that will have to be considered in evaluating the influence of changing social factors is related to the decrease in female dominance of mid-level health occupations. In addition to the increasing number of males being included in allied health and nursing programs, the changing role of women in health careers must also be considered. More and more women entering health careers are interested in pursuing these careers as a lifetime endeavor. This attitude is in sharp contrast with that of a generation ago when women tended to view their career as an interim between school and marriage.

In spite of these identifiable influences, however, society is changing so rapidly and needs are evolving so unpredictably that every effort must be made by all health professions to strive for identification of common curricular goals and career flexibility. If the health services industry is ever effectively to influence the health of our society, it is imperative that existing, restrictive legal and professional requirements and regulations be eliminated. Only then can individuals involved mold and develop their careers in ways that are personally rewarding and satisfying.

Education Trends. Many changes in the selection and education of physician's assistants reflect the evolution of our society in a very direct manner. Increasingly, as physician's assistants are accepted as members of the health care team, college graduates are seeking admission to the training programs. In spite of the expansion in the number of programs and the total accumulative enrollment, the quality of available candidates has continued to improve as they become more numerous. Also, whether or not related to the change in the characteristics of the potential candidates for the program, there is decreasing concern about the emphasis on extensive previous health care experience.

The year 1972 was particularly significant in that many programs for training physician's assistants became involved in a cooperative effort to develop core courses. This trend was both precipitated and marked by the formation of the Association of Physician Assistant Programs. The discourse associated with the formation of this organization reflected unity in direction while simultaneously being responsive to local and regional needs.

In spite of the great progress that has been made, there are still some rather significant differences in opinion between the validity of and emphasis on "task training" as compared with "health-Medical education." This difference of opinion is predominantly responsible for the differentiation in the educational process of MEDEX students and students enrolled in other physician's assistant programs.

During 1972 there was also increased emphasis by training programs on securing academic credit and granting various types of degrees. In all likelihood this trend will continue in the future. The emphasis on academic recognition is particularly interesting because the granting of academic credit and/or degrees makes little or no difference to the patient. In spite of this, the issue is of prime importance to the physician's assistant himself and to the academically indoctrinated physicians that serve as both their instructors and supervisors/employers. The importance of this issue reflects the organizational structure of the health services industry, which tends to equate performance and value with academic credentials. In spite of the apparent ludicrousness of this position, the granting of academic credit can be readily supported because of the associated professional and social importance. This will likely be increasingly true if the federal government becomes more directly involved in the delivery of health care services.

Problems. Many adverse factors loom on the horizon that could effectively retard the evolution and utilization of physician's assistants. Perhaps the most important of these is related to the fragmentation that currently exists between physician's assistants involved in the delivery of primary health care services and those involved in other more limited specialties. Likewise, the separation between physician's assistants and nurses functioning in an expanded role must be overcome if either or both are to be maximally effective.

Several problems related to the existing fragmentation within the concept itself have resulted from the lack of any early and effective leadership on the part of organized medicine. In retrospect it is difficult not to conclude that the AMA provided too little too late in the way of effective leadership. In so doing they encouraged the unorganized evolution of physician's assistants—a problem which they are now trying desperately to resolve. The problems associated with the inconsistent and uncoordinated curricula for specialist and generalist physician's assistants could have been eliminated had the AMA provided responsible leadership from the onset. One recent action (undertaken by the AMA in 1972 to deny categorically physicians employed by hospitals the opportunity to hire and utilize physician's assistants) appears to be totally inappropriate: available data from utilization studies indicate that the inpatient setting is one of the places where physician's assistants can be used most effectively.

CHALLENGES FOR THE FUTURE

In order for the physician's assistant to assume a logical, responsible and effective role in the delivery of health care services, the further evolution of the concept must be carefully coordinated by organized medicine, the many groups representing graduate physician's assistants, the federal government, the educational programs and organizations representing other health professions. In some way a forum of these groups must be established and maintained in a manner that can resolve existing group-interest differences and guide the future development of the profession. There are many obvious social problems that are either directly or indirectly related to the health and medical needs of our society which must be resolved within the purview of the health services industry unless it is to be subject to total governmental dominance.

The evolution of national standards that can have a built-in updating mechanism and thus assure the consumer of safety and quality is the most important single factor so far in establishing the lasting role of the physician's assistant.

The self-limited benefits associated with the protection of group interests and the generally antiquated mechanism under which health occupational groups function today must be eliminated. In their place an orderly, academic and professional mechanism for career progression with appropriate fiscal and social rewards must evolve. If physician's assistants are to remain a viable entity in the future, they must be able to fill whatever void exists between nursing and the traditional allied health occupations on one hand and physicians on the other.

It must be realized that physician's assistants represent a tremendous energy potential in the health services industry. As with nuclear energy, this human energy resource can be developed in a manner that can be either highly destructive or extremely beneficial. The major challenge that confronts the health services industry today is no different than the major challenge that confronts society as a whole. Very simply: we must resolve our differences at hand because our survival depends on our ability to "get it all together," and time is now a crucial factor.

NOTES

1. National Academy of Sciences, Washington, D.C., 1970.

2. John Braun, Office of Special Programs, Bureau of Health Manpower Education, National Institutes of Health, 9000 Rockville Pike, Bethesda, Md.

3. D. Robert Howard, Saul H. Jacobs and David E. Lewis, "Media Utilization and Needs in Physician's Assistant Programs and Related Medical-Health Education," Association of American Medical Colleges, 1973.

4. Alfred M. Sadler, Jr., Blair L. Sadler, and Ann A. Bliss, *The Physician's Assistant—Today and Tomorrow,* (New Haven: Yale University Press, 1972).

5. William Stanhope, "Eureka," *Journal of the American Academy of Physician's Associates* 3, No. 1 (January 1973).

6. *Proceedings of the Legal Conference on Physician's Assistants,* Duke University, 1968.

7. *Proceedings of the Second National Conference on Physician's Assistants,* Duke University, 1969.

8. *Proceedings of the First National Conference on Physician's Assistants,* Duke University, 1968; *Proceedings of the Third National Conference on Physician's Assistants,* Duke University, 1970.

9. *Proceedings of the Fourth National Conference on Physician's Assistants,* Duke University, 1972.

10. Suzanne Greenberg, Secretary-Treasurer, Association of Physician Assistant Programs, April, 1974.

11. *Essentials of an Approved Educational Program for the Assistant to the Primary Care Physician,* American Medical Association, December 1971.

12. National Association of Physicians' Assistants, 114 Liberty Street, Room 500, New York, N.Y.

OCCUPATIONAL THERAPY:

A PROFESSION IN TRANSITION

Jerry A. Johnson

Occupational therapy has been defined as "the art and science of directing man's participation in selected tasks to restore, reinforce and enhance performance, facilitate learning of those skills and functions essential for adaptation and productivity, diminish or correct pathology and to promote and maintain health. Reference to occupation in the title is in the context of man's goal-directed use of time, energy, interest and attention. Its fundamental concern is the development and maintenance of the capacity, throughout the life span, to perform with satisfaction to self and others those tasks and roles essential to productive living and to the mastery of self and the environment."[1]

The primary focus of occupational therapy is the development of adaptive skills and improved performance—not just in the realm of working for a living but in tasks and activities concerned with leisure, daily living and avocations, as well. It follows that the occupational therapist must be concerned with external or environmental barriers as well as biological or psychological problems which inhibit occupational performance. He or she must be equally alert to factors which influence or enhance performance.

Within this context of concerns, occupational therapists work with individuals whose abilities to cope with tasks of living are threatened or impaired by such problems as the aging process, physical injury or illness, psychological and/or social disability, chronic conditions, poverty and cultural differences, or deficits in perception-sensory-motor control or in cognitive, emotional or social development.

As a profession whose members increasingly are as concerned with prevention of disability and maintenance of health as with restoration of lost function, occupational therapy faces many challenges. These include: assessment, diagnosis, and intervention in all spheres of occupational performance; adapting the educational process to reflect traditional as well as newly-emerging areas of practice; gaining entry into and establishing new positions for expanded services in prevention and health maintenance in a society which continues to reward people for illness rather than encourage them to remain healthy.

They are also faced with establishing new relationships with physicians and other health professionals appropriate to professional goals and new environments in which occupational therapy may be practiced; dealing with a political system which grows increasingly complex as it integrates its support and standards with the delivery of health care systems; professional establishment and maintenance of standards for education, certification, and service; and the continued development of a body of knowledge, supported by research, to strengthen and expand the basic premises of occupational therapy.

Coping with these challenges is complicated by increasing external demands for health professionals to "speak as one unified body" rather than as separate professions.

For a small profession (approximately 16,000 members) any of these challenges could easily consume and require the total resources of that profession—both financial and human. However, occupational therapists have sought—and will continue to seek—answers and solutions in the belief that occupational therapy contributes a unique and necessary service devoted to the health of individuals.

EARLY HISTORY AND DEVELOPMENT

The National Society for the Promotion of Occupational Therapy was incorporated in March, 1917, at Clifton Springs,

New York, to further promote the concepts of occupational therapy.[2] These concepts were based on a theory (later postulated by Mary Reilly) that "man, through the use of his mind and body, can influence the state of his health."[3]

Members in the new association were to be selected from among those with previous training and successful experience in occupational therapy. The decision to admit to membership those who were already qualified insured that the founders and early members were persons sharing similar educational and occupational backgrounds. Consequently, the composition of the newly-formed organization was comprised of nurses, social workers, and individuals interested in health problems as well as in manual and industrial arts.[4]

The second major decision made by the founders was to establish a committee to develop "definite standards for the training of occupational therapists." As early as 1906, Miss Susan Tracy, superintendent of nurses at Adams Nervine Hospital in Boston, had standardized a scheduled course in occupational therapy and made it part of the curriculum in the training school for nurses.[5] Similar courses were established in other hospitals.

The purpose and philosophy of these early courses were articulated by Herbert Hall, M.D., of Deveraux Mansion, Marblehead, Massachusetts. Dr. Hall theorized that "manual and mental processes could be so linked to the remaining abilities of a patient that it would be possible to develop articles that had not only highly commercial value but the work could, and should, be correlated with curative exercises for special disabilities, administered by specially trained persons . . . who were knowledgeable with the medical arts and the fine arts."[6]

These efforts to create a solid professional basis for the practice of occupational therapy were given dramatic impetus by the sudden and burgeoning need for rehabilitation of wounded and disabled soldiers returning from World War I battlefields. Between 1918 and 1920, War Emergency and Civilian Service courses of three to four months duration were offered to train individuals to provide the needed therapy. By 1921 these courses had been extended to approximately twelve months in length, and most schools required an addi-

tional four months of either practical experience or clinical
training.

These early courses were offered by free-standing schools of
occupational therapy, by hospitals, and by colleges and universities.

Educational Standards Evolve. By 1923 the Teaching Methods
Committee had established standards setting forth the
minimum training requirements for occupational therapists.
A decade later the American Occupational Therapy Association (AOTA) (now renamed) became the first health profession to seek and obtain recognition of its educational process
by the American Medical Association. The minimum requirements of an acceptable course in occupational therapy in
1938 included 20 semester hours of theoretical subjects and
30 semester hours of technical instruction followed by 36
weeks of clinical training.   .

In the early 1940s all training programs became affiliated
with colleges or universities, and by 1947 the establishment of
educational standards and the process of accreditation was
full integrated into the functions of the national staff of the
AOTA.[7]

In the early versions of the *Essentials of an Accredited Educational Program in Occupational Therapy,*[8] the primary focus was
upon the course content, number of credits, and the physical
facilities of the occupational therapy school. The most recent
version, approved in October, 1972, reflects changes in the
educational process. It focuses on content and performance
of graduates, rather than on the less academic components of
the curriculum. This shift reflects a change in educational
philosophy and practice by recognizing that knowledge,
alone, is insufficient. The professional occupational therapist
must not only have knowledge but must be able to utilize that
knowledge for the accomplishment of identifiable and meas-
ureable goals or objectives.

Establishing Certifying Mechanisms. After educational standards were developed, physicians and other health professionals recommended in 1930 that a registration process for a

directory of qualified occupational therapists be established.
To be eligible for inclusion in the National Registry, occupational therapists had to graduate from an accredited school and complete one year of successful experience.[9] Support was given to the National Registry by leading physicians and hospital administrators "for the protection of hospitals and institutions from unqualified persons posing as occupational therapists."[10]

Later, the various schools of occupational therapy individually introduced essay style examinations for the purposes of further qualifying candidates for listing in the National Registry. In 1947, the American Occupational Therapy Association introduced an objective test to replace the essay type and to serve as the national registration examination.[11]

Through this process, the American Occupational Therapy Association developed its process of certifying occupational therapists at a national level. This national certifying mechanism has been maintained despite the trends and pressures created by many other health professions which have adopted the concept of state licensure. Whether the wisdom of this decision will prevail in the future is not known, for there are many external pressures on health professions to adopt state licensure, despite emerging suggestions by federal government officials to examine the alternatives of national or institutional certification.

In response to public concern about the policies of granting lifetime certification to members of professions (usually contingent only upon annual payment of certain fees), occupational therapists have developed a plan to work toward a process whereby all occupational therapists and certified occupational therapy assistants will have to regularly demonstrate their competence to practice in order to have their certification renewed.[12]

The adoption of this plan by the membership reflects a further shift in professional emphasis from inputs in the educational process to the knowledge and demonstrated performance of practising therapists. It reemphasizes the fact that the therapist must be able to utilize knowledge and skills in the attainment of identifiable goals in practice.

Occupational Therapy Assistants Are Recognized. The AOTA was one of the first organizations in the health professions to develop educational standards and recognition for assistant-level personnel. In 1958 the first set of training standards was adopted for occupational therapy assistants in psychiatry. These standards have since been revised to insure the education of occupational therapy assistants who can work in any of the major disability areas, and many of the training courses, originally offered in hospitals, have now been moved to junior or community colleges.[13]

Action taken by the Delegate Assembly in 1972 authorized the establishment of criteria whereby Certified Occupational Therapy Assistants can qualify to take the National Registration Examination, and the first was successfully completed in June, 1973. Having taken this step, assistants can become Registered Occupational Therapists without completing the traditional educational requirements.[14] Ex-military corpsmen who were trained as occupational therapy assistants in non-approved educational programs can now also qualify as Certified Occupational Therapy Assistants.

In 1973 the Delegate Assembly passed a resolution which, if accepted by the membership as a by-laws change, will permit certified occupational therapy assistants to be elected as Executive Board Members-at-Large.[15]

These initial steps taken by the occupational therapy profession offer persons trained at non-professional levels the opportunity to move upward within the profession.

Perhaps this review of the history of the development of occupational therapy will illustrate both the responsiveness of this profession to patient-client, societal, and professional needs and the way in which early decisions influenced the course of the profession's development.

OCCUPATIONAL THERAPY AS A PROFESSION IN TRANSITION

Occupational therapy, like many other health professions, is a profession in transition. Traditionally, the major concern of occupational therapy has been the restoration of persons who have incurred disability resulting from physical or psychological illness or injury, with a resulting loss in ability to perform. In fulfilling this commitment, occupational therapists have worked primarily in hospitals or other environments in which they have worked closely with physicians.

Now, however, changes in the traditional concepts of hospital utilization, the emergence of new types of health delivery centers, and evolving concepts about the contributions and role of occupational therapy are contributing to the status of occupational therapy as a profession in transition. Many hospitals are accepting only those patients with acute or serious conditions which require specialized medical tests or skilled medical supervision which cannot be provided in other settings, and the length of hospitalization is being reduced. Given this set of circumstances the occupational therapist's responsibility is to evaluate patients to determine if performance abilities have been impaired and if so, to what extent. The therapist can then instruct the patient and/or his family to carry out a planned treatment program, or a referral can be made for appropriate occupational therapy services after his discharge from the hospital.

In hospitals designed for long-term care and restoration or rehabilitation, occupational therapists continue to make major contributions in the evaluation, treatment, and training of individuals who have lost functional abilities as a result of such things as genetic defects, spinal cord injuries, cerebral vascular accidents, neurological disorders, arthritis, mental retardation or psychiatric problems.

The changing role of hospitals, as noted above, Medicare and other health and/or medical insurance legislation, spiraling costs of medical care, and the views occupational therapists have of their potential contributions in prevention and remediation, have all acted as catalysts to prompt occupational therapists to seek new environments in which to provide direct or indirect services. In this context, direct patient services include evaluation and treatment or training programs or assistance in the adaptation of living or work environments to enable clients to function independently or with minimal assistance from others. The occupational therapist might also provide indirect services by serving as a consultant to those providing direct patient or client services, as an educator who plans and/or provides continuing and advanced educational programs for therapists providing direct services, as a program coordinator, or as an administrator.

As occupational therapy developed, its concepts and practices were based upon the theory that gainful occupation of the mind *and* body in purposeful activity produced beneficial healing qualities as a result of the integration of psychological and physiological stimulation (thereby producing change in the pathological condition). Moreover, the patient participating in this process learned new skills and attitudes which enabled him to cope with, adapt to, or negotiate with, his environment. Because the occupational therapist worked with individuals in whom a healing process was occurring, he or she also functioned in close collaboration with the physician or appropriate medical specialist.

In this period of transition, many occupational therapists are transferring their knowledge and skills to delivery systems in which health care, rather than medical care, is provided. The characteristic which distinguishes the medical model is a pathological condition. In the health model, it is believed that man has some ability to control conditions which produce pathology and that he can thus influence or control his state of health. In other words, social or environmental conditions (e.g., poor sanitation, inadequate nutrition, polluted water), poor psychological conditions (e.g., a home environment which produces battered children), or personal habits (e.g., smoking, reckless driving, high accident rates in the home) are increasingly being linked to various pathological conditions. If such situations can be identified, and the suspected cause-effect relationship can be established, it is possible that many disabling or handicapping conditions can be prevented by changes in external conditions, by education, by early remediation, or by early treatment.[16]

Within the health model the occupational therapist's primary responsibility is to identify high-risk areas in which problems affecting the functional ability of individuals can be anticipated. Appropriate programming can then be developed based on need. For example, an occupational therapist working in a housing development identified a family on welfare. The father was working long hours on a low-paying job, the mother was mentally retarded, and there were two normal children. The mother did the grocery shopping but did not prepare meals or assist with other family activities. The therapist worked with her to teach her how to plan, prepare and serve nutritionally adequate meals, how to care for her house, and how to provide an environment in which the two children could have both structure and stimulation to support their intellectual development and normal growth.

In such situations the occupational therapist might work more closely with the social worker, the nurse, or the teacher than with the physician since the objective is to produce changes which, if ignored, may lead to pathological conditions. On the other hand, the occupational therapist in such situations might refer clients to the physician when it is suspected that problems in performance may arise from a medical condition. For this reason occupational therapists are frequently found in housing centers, in day-care centers, in nursery schools, in the public school system, in community centers, in "golden age" groups, and in vocational training schools.

With the continued development of a body of knowledge of and about occupational therapy, the roles and contributions of occupations as therapeutic media in occupational therapy have assumed greater significance and importance. For example, in the child development and evaluation centers established by the Public Health Service, the information gained from the occupational therapy evaluations of the child as he engages in a selected occupation often is of prime importance in differentiating among mental retardation, autism, or perceptual deficits. The appropriate diagnosis can be critical to a child and his family in that it can strongly influence expectations that many people (e.g., health professionals, the family, teachers) have for the child. It also may determine whether or not a remedial or treatment program is planned for the child. Occupation as utilized in occupational therapy requires some degree of physiological, psychological, cognitive, and social integration within the individual; deficits in any one of those components, or resulting from problems affecting two or more components, may not appear in evaluation procedures directed only toward discrete problems, i.e., physical development. Thus, the ability or inability to perform given activities becomes a valuable diagnostic tool.

Occupational therapists are now utilizing more than arts and crafts in their programming—another aspect of change in recent years. The appropriate use of any occupation depends upon the needs of the client/patient, the purposes or goals to be fulfilled through the occupational therapy program, and the developmental level of the individual in social, cognitive, emotional, and sensory-perceptual-motor spheres. In most instances, the occupation utilized in occupational therapy involves the patient/client in a participatory-learning process. Thus in working with small children the activities to be employed might be toys, games, or exercises which stimulate the central nervous system and which enable the child to use his body more appropriately, while he also learns to manipulate objects in his phsyical environment. For an adolescent, the appropriate activities might be those relating to the development of social skills, an improved self-image, and exploration of possible vocational interests or abilities.

Occupation, particularly that resulting in a new skill or a finished product, provides direct feedback to the individual about himself, his level of performance or competence, his abilities, and his value to himself or to others. It is frequently through successful performance and occupation that individuals gain a feeling of mastery over their environment, thereby giving up feelings of helplessness about their inability to influence or affect the environment in which they live. Inability to perform satisfactorily tends to produce feelings of helplessness, and occupational therapy's goals include those of enabling the individual to cope with, adapt to, or negotiate with the environment in which he lives, thereby reducing his sense of helplessness.

In the past, occupational therapy might not have been necessary for many individuals with performance deficits (with the exception of those who were catastrophically disabled by illness or injury), for they could be accommodated by an agrarian or rural society in which manual skills were important and valued. However, a technological society requires and values verbal and cognitive skills as well as the capacity for abstract thought, logic, and analysis. People who lack or have not had the opportunity to develop these skills and abilities easily become failures. Even household items, which earlier could be repaired by someone with the ability to handle tools and with basic understanding of mechanics or electrical design, are now made to be replaced when they break. Thus, the average individual is deprived of the sense of value, worth, or competence which could be gained from his mastery over objects in his environment.

Man's need to feel that he is able to manage and control events in the environment partially explains the popular movement in the United States toward development of hobbies or the "do-it-yourself" syndrome. However, even these alternatives are unavailable for those who lack adequate financial resources. Further, hobbies provide gratification to the participating individual but they do not necessarily provide the sense of value obtained by making a contribution to or being needed by others.

In summary, occupational therapy is a profession in transition. Its original goals were to help individuals regain functional skills or performance capacities which had been lost or impaired as a result of illness, injury, or congenital defect. Now, however, our society contains individuals who are disabled or handicapped not only by illness and injury but because they cannot function adequately in a technological society. Consequently, occupational therapists are expanding into new environments to help prevent disability and maintain health by applying their knowledge and skills about occupational performance to new client populations.

These changes have particular relevance for occupational therapy educators, for they require not only a new educational philosophy but significant curriculum changes involving cognitive, affective, and experiential learning.

To accomplish and implement these changes, the Council on Education of the American Occupational Therapy Association is in the process of reviewing and revising the *Essentials of an Accredited Educational Program for the Occupational Therapist*. This will help insure that educational standards and objectives are consistent with the direction and practice of the profession. Greater latitude in selection of clinical sites for affiliations is also encouraged to enable students to practice occupational therapy in a variety of environments and with persons who have or may develop occupational dysfunctions resulting from psychological, biological, or sociological causes.

Such fundamental changes in curricula and affiliation patterns have far-reaching implications, for they require that occupational therapy educators identify, articulate, integrate, and transmit the body of knowledge which is the science of occupational therapy.

Earlier models of education have suggested that the disciplines of medicine, psychology, and biology were the foundations for occupational therapy theory. The evolution of occupational therapy, as presented here, implies that there is a body of theory unique to occupational therapy which utilizes principles from other disciplines. Consequently, an occupational therapy student need not study pathology as an end in itself but as a means to understanding occupational dysfunction and the implications for treatment or remediation. Further, the occupational therapy student must have understanding of health as a concept, a goal, and a condition, each of which is influenced by purposeful occupation.

In this newer framework, the occupational therapist is primarily concerned with the meaning of occupation, the assessment of occupational performance and behavior, the identification of occupational dysfunction, and the means by which intervention can occur to facilitate and enhance effective and satisfying occupational performance.

As occupational therapy educators previously designed course content for treatment of specific disability or pathological conditions, they will now have to design content related to the areas of occupational performance. In essence the core of occupational therapy education becomes occupational therapy itself, whereas previously the core centered on conditions or diagnostic categories with which occupational therapists worked or the biological, psychological, and medical sciences.

In summary, the changes pose many challenges for educators and practitioners alike as they review and revise the components of occupational therapy education.

Major Issues Confronting the Profession

Just as occupational therapy clients are confronted with the demands of a technological society, the occupational therapy profession must also deal with ever-changing external forces seeking change among health professions and in the health delivery system. These external forces may consist of 1) governmental agencies or consumer groups seeking to regulate health delivery; 2) private agencies or larger organizations seeking to regulate educational standards, to evaluate such standards, or to become the "unified voice" for all health disciplines; and/or 3) legislators who establish standards and authorize payment for the provision of health services.

In addition to dealing with external forces, the occupational therapy profession is also concerned with issues such as educational philosophy, content, and directions; maintenance of professional competence to practice; facilitating the movement of therapists into new areas of practice where there is need; and advancement and testing of the theories of occupational therapy.

Certification and Licensure. The American Occupational Therapy Association in its early development adopted a certifying process which was controlled by the profession and referred to nationally as registration for Registered Occupational Therapists and as certification for Occupational Therapy Assistants. As licensure became a more common practice for health professionals, the profession evaluated and compared its national registration system to state licensure. It then adopted a position strongly in support of national certification.

Licensure was viewed as restricting the mobility of therapists, inhibiting the movement of the professional prac-

tice into new areas or environments, and as limiting opportunities for either upward mobility within the profession or
entry into the profession by any alternative means. There was
also concern about the possible loss of control over the licensing process with a resulting lowering of standards for service.

Basically, the above rationale continues to have strong
merit, but external forces—in a drive to improve the overall
quality of health care, to reduce the cost of such care, and to
insure that health care is responsive to the needs of consumers
rather than protective of professionals—are challenging all
existing certifying mechanisms. Proponents of national certification are advocating studies which might lead to a national
certification system for all health professions. They argue that
it will insure consistent standards of care, enable practitioners
to move without difficulty into areas with demonstrated personnel shortages, and permit existing health professions to
expand the scope of their services without the necessity of
having to resort to the development of new professional or
occupational groups to fulfill narrow specializations.

Proponents of state licensure, on the other hand, suggest
that it can exert more direct control over the quality of care
provided and the maintenance of standards by practicing
health professions than can other systems. Furthermore, if
manpower shortages exist in a given geographical area, it is
conceivable that the state licensure system could grant licenses
to individuals only if they practice in designated geographical
areas. Massachusetts, in its governmental reorganization
plan, has proposed an eight-member regulatory board which
will include 3 health professionals (one of whom must be a
physician) and 5 lay persons. This board will have the powers
of licensure and cost regulation, among other powers.[17] Thus
it is conceivable that the professions could lose their responsibility for establishment and maintenance of standards for
certification.

Proponents of institutional licensure suggest that the most
effective and efficient method of licensure is to have the major
responsibility rest with the institutions providing care. This
system may be the most closely related to the supply-demand
concept of capitalistic institutions in that there is an assump-

tion that if an institution provides services which the public wants, the public will pay for those services. Therefore, it is to the institution's advantage to insure that its personnel are qualified and provide a quality of care at least consistent with public demand. The major disadvantage of this system, however, is that theoretically an institution could by-pass professional certification, thereby employing and licensing whomever it wished.

Problems created by the current state licensure system may indeed serve as catalysts to move professions utilizing other certifying mechanisms to adopt state licensure, despite its disadvantages. For example, under some forms of state and federal legislation, state licensure is necessary for a professional to be reimbursed for services directly as a member of an independent health profession without having to meet the requirements of referral by and supervision of a physician. Secondly, some state and/or federal institutions refuse to acknowledge professional standards for certification and will employ or permit employment of persons who are not recognized by the profession, unless state licensure exists. Even in this instance federal institutions are not bound by state licensure.

While factors governing future certifying mechanisms are ambiguous at this time, it appears that any certifying process will be concerned with initial entry into the profession, maintenance of competence to continue practicing throughout one's lifetime (or until retirement), and mechanisms by which recognition is awarded. Moreover, the processes of utilization review, public audit, peer review, and other evaluation mechanisms seem likely to proliferate and expand. Of concern to many health professionals is the question of whether each profession will be responsible for peer review or whether they may be evaluated by physicians, the lay public, or others who may not have adequate understanding of the profession.[18]

It well may be necessary for the occupational therapy profession to reevaluate its stand on national registration and licensure to determine what action it must take in the face of external pressures. As with other small professional associations, however, (small in both numbers of members and their earning power) the decisions made by external bodies or forces around this issue may well determine the fate and destiny of those organizations in terms of whether they retain the power and authority to make major decisions about educational standards, accreditation of schools, certification of personnel, and standards of practice (as well as areas in which such practice may be conducted). If small organizations lose the power of professional decision-making in these areas, the role of professional associations and of the professions themselves will have to be seriously reconsidered.

Government Affairs and Occupational Therapy. Government affairs are of prime concern to occupational therapists today in that government has considerable influence over the standards for and delivery of services and the reimbursement policies for those services. Historically, few individual occupational therapists have actively participated in lobbying to influence legislation, supporting elected officials or candidates for elective office, or other political activities. However, it is increasingly necessary for professional disciplines to be written into legislation and into the implementing regulations. In moving to participate more actively in dealing with external forces, the AOTA has a firm foundation in its highly organized and centralized national organization structure. However, its present weakness is that it does not also have a consistently strong state or regional organizational structure which could easily be equipped to deal with the decreasing centralization of the federal government and the increasing involvement of regional offices in the area of health delivery. This weakness is intensified by the fact that many occupational therapists have traditionally demonstrated little interest in assuming leadership roles or in attempting to influence external matters. Consequently, the profession is faced with the need to strengthen its organizational structure at the regional and local levels and to recruit and prepare therapists for leadership positions at the same time.

It is obvious that occupational therapy's problems in relation to governmental affairs and external forces may have bearing on ultimate decisions about certification as they evolve through the legislative process.

Funding Occupational Therapy Services. Generally, funding for occupational therapy services was not a serious problem when they were provided in traditional medical settings or were closely identified with medical or rehabilitation models of service. However, in its transitional role and with the present trend of hospitals to reduce or eliminate services not directly related to primary medical care, methods of funding must receive greater attention.

The American public has not yet made a commitment to support preventive health services, and occupational therapy is not yet widely recognized as a profession which can make contributions in some of the non-medical settings such as school systems, community centers, housing developments, and departments of human resources. Moreover, within the concept of health maintenance organizations and health care services for which individuals are reimbursed by insurance and third party providers, there is a reluctance to recognize occupational therapy as a reimbursable service.

These are all serious problems for occupational therapists, particularly in that members of the profession and the professional association have not devoted adequate attention to any basic marketing or public education concepts which would bring the value of occupational therapy services to public attention. For numerous reasons occupational therapists generally are most content when working with patients or clients and have overlooked the necessity to attend to external matters which will insure their continuing services. This attitude is a hold-over from the era when all occupational therapy services were provided by written prescriptions from the physicians and when physicians took more active responsibility to assure the continuing availability of occupational therapy services.

In comparison to medicine with its scientific approach, occupational therapists have continued to utilize a humanistic approach to patient care. While one cannot challenge the value of the humanistic approach, it does not meet the criteria now being established for reimbursable medical or health care services.

It is becoming increasingly apparent that occupational therapists must give serious consideration to the potential sources of funding for their services and to changes which may have to be made within the profession if therapists are to qualify for reimbursement. This issue cannot be considered apart from the issues of certification, legislation, government affairs, and other external forces, because they are all interrelated.

Relationships with Other Major Health Professions. One of the occupational therapy profession's greatest challenges is that of finding and establishing appropriate relationships with those health professions with which it shares similar interests and concerns. There is mounting pressure—particularly within the government, which is reflected through actions in other groups—for health professions to speak with a unified voice rather than to press for their individual interests. This has provided an impetus for some groups or organizations to seek to become the spokesmen for many of the smaller health professions.

The disadvantages and weaknesses inherent in this action are that professional identity—already a problem among occupational therapists—is further reduced, and groups of health professionals are "lumped" together without concern for the nature of their professional roles and contributions, their educational requirements, or their relationships to physicians or clients. Too frequently, the interests of the primary "sponsoring" body, rather than the interests and concerns of the individual health professions, are protected. Finally, in the decision-making process, the influence of the small, individual health professions is reduced or neutralized by the many and varied committees through which decisions and policies must pass. At each step, the voices of the smaller organizations are diluted and become less effective.

Many groups have been formed to speak collectively for the health professions (the American Society of Allied Health Professions, the Coalition of Independent Health Professions, the American Medical Association's Advisory Committee for Allied Health Education, and the National Health Council). Yet none has really moved into a position of strong, accepted leadership.

There·are many needs which such a group could fill to provide a forum for planning, to reduce competition among health professionals, to seek solutions to common problems, and to provide mutual support and assistance in improving health services. However, for such groups or coalitions to be effective, ways must be found to enable the leaders of the professions concerned to participate in the final decision-making processes or to be represented by persons who share and/or understand their concerns. The groups seeking to become the spokesmen for groups of health professions do not generally include representatives of unions, business, insurance companies, or consumers in the decision-making bodies, so the decisions which are made most frequently are for the protection of the professions themselves. An exception is the National Health Council, and it has not yet shown any interest in performing this role.

It is going to be increasingly necessary for health professions to form coalitions so that they can address and resolve common or shared concerns, but how this will be done is not yet known. Perhaps the need for such coalitions may not be evident to many of the health professions, particularly those which have been more successful so far in terms of dealing with legislation, funding, and other mechanisms which act to insure their survival. Conversely, for those organizations which have not resolved issues related to their basic economic security, joining a coalition may present difficulties in that joint decisions usually require each of the participants to know just what can be negotiated and on what issues one must take a firm stand.[19]

In summary, occupational therapists need to make more concerted efforts to determine how they can best respond to the demands of external forces, where and on what issues they want to exercise initiative—particularly in relation to external forces—and through what means they can achieve economic security and professional survival.

Education and Occupational Therapy. Education of students
who will become occupational therapists has been one of the
major activities in which the professional association has been
involved, and a major portion of both human and economic
resources within the profession has been allocated to the
educational process. This has resulted in the preparation of
knowledgeable clinicians who enter occupational therapy; but
it has done little to support therapists as they acquire invaluable experience which enriches their knowledge, skills, and
potential contributions to clients. The profession as a whole
must become more supportive of clinicians and should act to
promote the creation of positions for clinical specialists and
researchers.

At present, for occupational therapists to advance professionally within the health care system, individuals most frequently have to move into administration, teaching, or into
another professional discipline. Thus, the profession is deprived of those individuals who are most knowledgeable and
experienced and who could be responsible for studies and
research from which textbooks are written and upon which
appropriate bodies of knowledge are developed.

The membership of the AOTA has voiced strong support
for the concept of establishing and maintaining systems which
will insure that occupational therapists maintain their competency to practice. This decision suggests that priorities must be
re-examined so that there is a better balance of educational
resources as they are allocated to initial preparation of clinicians and continuing or advanced education for experienced
clinicians.

In an indirect fashion, this decision may have been an
extremely wise one to make, for if knowledgeable and experienced therapists remain in the profession, they may be more
willing to exert leadership roles in moving the professional
association to make some of the basic professional decisions
which need to be made.

Young clinicians, generally speaking, devote their energies
to the care of patients and clients. The more experienced
clinicians who remain in the profession are more aware that
the ability to provide quality services is related both to the

knowledge and skill of the individual therapist and to the external conditions which influence the delivery of such services.

Again, significant changes will be required in the philosophy and design of basic professional education programs. An illustration of such changes is demonstrated in the curriculum outline (pp. 222-23) and course descriptions (abstracted) prepared through the collaborative efforts of clinical and academic occupational therapists for Towson State College, Baltimore, Maryland.[20]

COURSE DESCRIPTIONS

Dynamics of Occupation in Human Living (2)
The concept of occupation as man's use of time, energy and attention as a force in normal human behavior. Fundamentals applicable to personal development and community living. The positive and negative forces of human participation in typical daily living experiences.

Impact of Occupational Therapy
On Contemporary Society (1)
The study of occupational therapy as one of the health professions, types of services provided, types of clients served, work opportunities, and relationship with other professional disciplines are covered. One-half day per week for 6-8 weeks are spent in field observation of occupational therapy practice.

Human Growth and Development (4)
A study of physical, perceptual, cognitive, emotional and social growth processes and age related developmental tasks from birth to old age. The impact of stress (emotional and physical), trauma and disease on normal development and wellness is included.

Dynamics of Occupation in Health Advocacy (2)
A study of the use of occupation as a force in the equilibrium of health. Primary emphasis will be on the role and type of occupation in age appropirate groups (play, education, em-

Occupational Therapy

First Year

First Semester

Human Anatomy & Physiology I	4
General Psychology	3
Introduction to Sociology	3
Dynamics of Occupation in Human Living with Impact of Occupational Therapy on Contemporary Society	3
English	3
Elective	(2)
	16-18

Second Semester

Human Anatomy & Physiology II	4
Human Growth & Development with Physical & Social Module	4
Mental Hygiene	3
Dynamics of Occupation in Health Advocacy	2
English	3
Elective	(2)
	16-18

Second Year

Third Semester

Causes of Occupational Dysfunction	4
Dynamics of Occupation in Health Management	3-5
Dynamics of Occupation in Illness	6-7
Physical Education	1
Elective	(2)
	14-19

Fourth Semester

Current Issues of Occupational Therapy in the Health Care Delivery System	3
Current Health Problems	3
Field Experience I	4
Elective	3
Elective	3 (5)
	16-18

THIRD YEAR

Fifth Semester

Logic	3
Analysis of Human Motion	3
Statistics (Basic or Behavioral)	3
Small Groups	3
Dynamics of Occupational Therapy	3
Elective	1 (3)
	16-18

Sixth Semester

Tests & Measurements	3
Personality	3
Economics of Health	3
Management of the Dynamics of Occupational Therapy	6
Elective	1 (3)
	16-18

FOURTH YEAR

Seventh Semester

Field Experience	7
Field Experience	7
Quantification in the Dynamics of Occupational Therapy	1-3
Field Experience (Optional)	(3)
	15-20

Eighth Semester

Occupational Therapy Organization Administration and Teaching	3
Synthesis of Occupational Therapy Theory & Practice	2
Exploration in the Dynamics of Occupation	2-3
Electives	9 (11)
	16-19

ployment, retirement) relevant to differing societies/
subcultures and their accepted health norms. Individual and
societal adjustment to the work ethic and acceptance of defi-
cient behavior is included.

Causes of Performance Dysfunction (4)
The major types of injuries, diseases and environmental conditions amenable to occupational therapy are studied. Etiol-
ogy, biological-psychological-social processes, medical precautions, prognosis for recovery and functional loss are covered with a view towards occupational therapy treatment
potential and rehabilitation principles. Classroom instruction will be augmented by actual and video case presentations
as available from medical, psychiatric, child development and
other community resources.

Dynamics of Occupation in Health Management (3-5)
Fundamentals of task analysis for successful occupational
performance and task achievement. Self-care, games, academic and work tasks, and creative activities are examined
for requisite cognitive-motor schemes and affective components. Effects of familial and cultural stimulation are compared with effects of sensory and socioeconomic deprivation.
Students will be expected to contribute their analysis of tasks
indigenous to most environs, e.g., self-care and domestic arts,
as well as contribute from their background in special skills
among the variety of media used to develop, maintain or
restore function.

Dynamics of Occupation in Illness (6-7)
Analysis of the dynamics of occupation in the presence of
pathology. The perimeters of its application, the precautions,
the crises to be avoided or overcome in its use will be studied as
an influence upon human behavior. The distortion of normal
dynamics and theory in the application of occupation in the
spectrum of faulty development, illness, and disability will be
explored. Emphasis will be on the problem solving process of
client evaluation and data gathering, data analysis and program planning, communications, and program implementa-

tion appropriate to the occupational therapy assistant. Independent practice will be arranged for students needing or desiring additional clinical/laboratory study.

*Current Issues of Occupational Therapy
in the Health Care Delivery System (3)*
This course is correlated with concurrent field experience in the delivery of occupational therapy services. Institutional versus community based and home care services are reviewed. Case finding, referral, communication and supervisory systems are challenged within the context of team and authoritarian structures. Apparent conflicting treatment frames of reference are analyzed for common generic elements and congruence. Professional ethics, etiquette and legal implications are included.

Field Experience I (4)
Field Experience II (4)
A selected period of 4 to 5 weeks each full-time supervised field application with the opportunity to provide occupational services to clients of both sexes, varying levels of chronicity and range of developmental ages. By combination between Field Experience I and II the student will need to insure that the field education includes a variety of learning experiences in physical and psychosocial function.

Field Experience III (4)
A selected period of 4-5 weeks full-time supervised field application to meet the special interests and experiences of the individual student. Extension of Field Experience I or II may be selected or experience in specialized areas may be arranged, e.g., experience in mental retardation, pediatrics, geriatrics, community health.

Analysis of Human Motion (3)
Optimal integration of body systems for normal function. Primary focus on neurophysiology, endocrinology, and musculoskeletal function. Motor and imagery constructs in learning are included.

Dynamics of Occupational Therapy (3)
Dynamics of occupation in client evaluation and program planning with goal approximation for landmarking of change in client behavior. The projection of long and short term goals, the projection of judgment to determine client-appropriate goals, the type and amount of service required to achieve them, identification of institutional, family and community resources and of factors intruding upon success.

Management of the Dynamics of Occupational Therapy (6)
Selected sequencing and guidance of applied dynamics, analysis of their effects and projection of the outcome of continued or altered application of principles in specific service and in support of client need. Cerkships assignments will be concerned with evaluation of clients, refinement of goal setting, appraisal of client progress and of clinician or consultant performance, discreet phasing of frequency and amount of treatment or of daily regimen change indicated or contraindicated for the use of occupational therapy in client management. (Students with prior experience in client evaluation and application of occupational therapy at the therapist level may challenge the clerkship objectives of this course through evidence of prior field learning and examination.)

Field Experience IV (7)
Field Experience V (7)
A selected period of three to four months each full time field application and supervised experience with the opportunity to provide occupational therapy services to clients of both sexes, varying levels of chronicity and range of developmental stages. By combination with other field experience the student will need to insure that the field education includes a variety of learning experiences in perceptual-cognitive-motor development, psychosocial function, and physical function in both institutional and community delivery systems.

Quantification in the Dynamics of
Occupational Therapy (1-3)
Independent study exploring the forces of occupation in the

treatment of pathology and as a health influence upon client behavior, and upon the maintenance of an environment supportive of health, for acceptable quantification of occupational therapy.

Field Experience VI (optional) (3)
A selected period of two or three months for field experience in a specialized area, e.g., mental retardation, cerebral palsy, blind and visually impaired, child psychiatry, adolescent psychiatry, special education, pediatrics, geriatrics, public health, drug abuse, penology, juvenile delinquency.

Occupational Therapy Organization,
Administration and Teaching (3)
The focus of this course is on principles of organization, administration, personnel management and development in occupational therapy service programs. It includes systems analysis, program planning, budgetary planning, space and facilities planning, staff selection and supervision, communication and record systems, cost analysis and cost effectiveness, medico-legal considerations and programs for professional staff and student development. Students will be expected to supply critiques of prior organizations with which they have had experience.

Synthesis of Occupational Therapy Theory and Practice (2)
This discussion style recapitulation provides the students with opportunities to relate prior education to problems and experiences they encounter in field experience.

Exploration in the Dynamics of Occupation (1-3)
Independent research in the forces of occupation to identify new factors toward enhancement of the basic knowledge of such forces and their impact upon contemporary society and potential impact for change in societal living habits to support optimum health.

In reviewing the above curriculum, it can be seen that its emphasis is on occupational therapy as it utilizes and focuses on occupation, occupational assessment, identification of occupational dysfunction, and appropriate intervention to prevent or treat potential or real dysfunction.

A curriculum such as this no longer separates therapists by the diagnostic groups with whom they are concerned. Rather, it identifies the core and foundation of occupational therapy and identifies the system around which basic professional education for all occupational therapy students can be designed. It implies that graduate education for occupational therapists (beyond initial certification) might focus on one or more of the applied sciences—e.g., biological, medical, psychological, sociological—or specializations which would facilitate the development of highly competent clinicians within the profession.

Through the conscious development and support of such clinicians by the profession, there should follow an increase in research and theory as they relate to the science of occupational therapy.

SUMMARY

Occupational therapy is a profession in transition which has unique and valuable contributions to make to individuals who have lost (or are threatened with the potential loss of) ability to function as a result of illness, injury, disability, social-psychological-environmental conditions, or habits which inhibit or are detrimental to their ability to function independently in fulfilling their tasks of daily living.

Members of the occupational therapy profession have tended to focus on client services rather than on any of the external conditions which are now exerting considerable influence on delivery of health services. Consequently, occupational therapists must begin to determine how they wish to deal with these external forces and to recognize the importance and necessity of making such decisions. Throughout the history of occupational therapy, its members have adapted to changing conditions and consumer needs. Thus, there is every reason to believe that the present challenges will be met and eventually resolved as the profession increases its contributions to the health delivery system as well as to the patients and the clients that it serves.

NOTES

1. J. A. Johnson (ed.), "Report of the Task Force on Social Issues," *American Journal of Occupational Therapy* 26 (1972):348.

2. E. D. Slagle, "Occupational Therapy," *The Trained Nurse and Hospital Review* 1938: p. 376.

3. Mary Reilly, "Occupational Therapy Can Be One of the Great Ideas of 20th Century Medicine," *AJOT* 16 (1962):2.

4. Slagle, p. 380.

5. S. E. Tracy, *Invalid Occupations*, (Boston: Whitcomb and Barrows, 1910).

6. Slagle, p. 378.

7. "Developmental Changes in Occupational Therapy" (unpublished paper) (1952), American Occupational Therapy Association.

8. "Essentials of an Accredited Educational Program in Occupational Therapy," American Medical Association and American Occupational Therapy Association.

9. Slagle, p. 380.

10. "Developmental Changes."

11. "Developmental Changes."

12. *Delegate Assembly Resolution* 300-71, AOTA.

13. M. W. Crampton, "Educational Upheaval for Occupational Therapy Assistants," *AJOT* 21 (1967):317.

14. *Delegate Assembly Resolution* 246-70, AOTA.

15. *Delegate Assembly Resolution* 356-73, AOTA.

16. Johnson, "Report of the Task Force," pp. 349-351.

17. Massachusetts House Bill No. 620, (1973).

18. J. A. Johnson, "Government and the Professions: Setting Public Standards Through Private Organizations—Future Directions for Licensing, Certifying and Reviewing Performance," *AJOT* 27 (1973):257.

19. F. S. Cromwell, "The President's Address," *AJOT* 26 (1972):367.

20. "A Proposed Undergraduate Program in Occupational Therapy," Towson State College, Baltimore, Maryland, May 1973. (Supported in part by National Institute of Health Planning Grant #1 D12 AH 00464-01 from the Division of Allied Health Manpower.)

LIST OF CONTRIBUTORS

RUTH M. FRENCH, M.A., MT (ASCP), is associate dean, School of Associated Medical Sciences, and professor of clinical laboratory sciences at the University of Illinois at the Medical Center. She is a member of the Review Board of the National Accrediting Agency for Clinical Laboratory Sciences, and of the Board of Trustees of the ASMT Education & Research Fund, Inc., serving as its chairman in 1972-73. Ms. French is a member of the editorial boards of the *American Journal of Medical Technology* and the *Journal of Allied Health*. She is the author of *Nurse's Guide to Diagnostic Procedures* (now in its third edition), and *Dynamics of Health Care* (now in its second edition).

JOSEPH HAMBURG, M.D., has been dean of the College of Allied Health Professions, University of Kentucky, since 1966. He is also professor of allied health education research and holds the joint appointment of professor of medicine and of community medicine. He was in private practice for eleven years in Connecticut. Dr. Hamburg is a founding institutional member (1966) of the American society of Allied Health Professions and was the society's president in 1969 and 1970. He is a member of the board of directors of the National Health Council and serves as an allied health consultant to the U.S. Air Force.

JOHN W. HEIN, D.M.D., Ph.D., is director of the Forsyth Dental Center in Boston; its three divisions are the Forsyth Institute for Research and Advanced Study in Dentistry, the Forsyth School for Dental Hygienists and the Forsyth Dental Infirmary. Dr. Hein has divided his interest and his career among dental education, dental research, organized dentistry and industry. He was formerly chairman of the Department of Dentistry and Dental Research, University of Rochester (1952-55) and was dean of Tufts University School of Dental Medicine from 1959 to 1962. A former president of the Massachusetts Dental Society (1964), Dr. Hein is currently the deans' representative to the board of trustees of the society. He serves as consultant to several companies.

DENNIS ROBERT HOWARD, M.D., is chief of the division of graduate education in family medicine and associate professor of community health and family medicine, University of Florida. At Duke University (1968-72) he was first medical director, then director, of the physician's associate program. Dr. Howard was in private practice in family medicine for several years in Wisconsin. He is a past president of the American Registry of Physician's Associates, Inc. (1970-72) and has written extensively on the subject of the physician's associate.

MARCELINE E. JAQUES, Ph.D., is professor and director of the Rehabilitation Counselor Education Program, Department of Counselor Education, State University of New York at Buffalo, and a clinical professor in the School of Health Related Professions there. She is a former executive director of the Black Hills Rehabilitation Center in Rapid City, South Dakota, and a former staff member of the National Society for Crippled Children. Dr. Jaques is chairman of the board of directors of the Center for Human Services Training, Inc., New York State Department of Mental Hygiene. She is past president of the American Rehabilitation Counseling Association (1966-68) and current president of the Council of Rehabilitation Counselor Educators. She is a former member of the editorial board of *The Personnel and Guidance Journal* and current editor of the *Rehabilitation Counseling Bulletin*.

JERRY A. JOHNSON, Ed.D., OTR, is professor and associate dean for academic affairs, Sargent College of Allied Health Professions, Boston University. She was formerly professor and director, Center for Allied Health Instructional Personnel, University of Florida (1971-72) and served as executive director of the Alton, Ill., Easter Seal Society (1957-59). Ms. Johnson is president of the American Occupational Therapy Association and past president of the Massachusetts Association of Occupational Therapy. She was a member of the Massachusetts Governor's Task Force on Training and Manpower in Mental Health (1964-65). Ms. Johnson is the author of numerous published articles in the field of occupational therapy.

DAVID E. LEWIS, M.A., assistant professor at the University of Florida, is associate director of the Physician's Assistant Program, College of Medicine, University of Florida/Santa Fe Community College in Gainesville, Florida. From 1968 to 1972 he held a similar position at Duke University Medical School where he was also an associate in the Department of Community Health Sciences.

SAMUEL P. MARTIN, M.D., is professor of community medicine both in the School of Medicine of the University of Pennsylvania and in the Health Care Unit of its Wharton School of Finance and Commerce. Former faculty appointments include Duke University (1949-56) and University of Florida (1956-71). He was a visiting professor at the London School of Hygiene and Tropical Medicine, University of London, in 1970 and at the Harvard Medical School and John Fitzgerald Kennedy School of Government, Harvard University, from 1969 to 1971. Dr. Martin has held varied positions as administrator and consultant in the medical and health fields. He was a research fellow of the American College of Physicians at Rockefeller Institute for Medical Research. Dr. Martin is the author or co-author of almost a hundred published articles.

DARREL J. MASE, Ph. D., joined the staff of the University of Florida in 1950 as coordinator of the Florida Center of Clinical Services, professor of speech, psychology and education, and is at the university at the present time. In 1958, he became dean of the College of Health Related Professions in the J. Hillis Miller Health Center. At present he is dean emeritus and professor in that college. Since 1971, he has worked in the health systems research division and he also has an appointment in the division of community health and family medicine in the department of medicine in the College of Medicine. Dr. Mase has devoted much of his career to working in behalf of the mentally retarded and physically handicapped. He served on President Kennedy's Panel on Mental Retardation as well as many other national and international boards. He was the first president (1967-68) of the Association of Schools of Allied Health Professions (now the American Society of Allied Health Professions).

EDMUND D. PELLEGRINO, M.D., is chancellor of the Medical Units, vice president for health affairs and professor of medicine and medical humanities, University of Tennessee. He was formerly vice president for health sciences, State University of New York Medical Center at Stony Brook (1966-73). Dr. Pellegrino was chairman of the AMA Advisory Committee on Education for the Allied Health Professions and Services, Council on Medical Education (1967-73) and also chairman of the AMA Committee on Nursing. He serves on the editorial boards of *The Pharos of Alpha Omega, American Family Physician,* as chairman of *Journal of Medical Education,* and as editor-in-chief of the *Journal of Medicine and Philosophy.* Dr. Pellegrino is author or co-author of two hundred published papers in the fields of science, medicine education and philosophy. He serves as a consultant to civilian and veterans' hospitals.

J. WARREN PERRY, Ph.D., is dean of the School of Health Related Professions and professor of health sciences administration at State University of New York at Buffalo. On a recent leave of absence he served as director of a study of allied health education for the American Association of Community and Junior Colleges. He is a former director of continuing education, orthopaedic surgery, Northwestern University Medical School (1956-59). From 1960 to 1966 Dr. Perry was deputy assistant commissioner of the Vocational Rehabilitation Administration in the federal Department of Health, Education and Welfare. He is editor of *Journal of Allied Health*, past president of American Society of Allied Professions, and a member of the Institute of Medicine, National Academy of Sciences.

A. BRADLEY SOULE, M.D., Sc.D., F.A.C.R., is a consultant in radiology and professor emeritus at the University of Vermont College of Medicine. He served as professor and then chairman of the radiology department there from 1936 to 1970. Dr. Soule's leadership in the growth and development of radiologic technology over the past half century won him life membership in the American Society of Radiologic Technologists. He is a former trustee and president of the American Registry of X-ray Technicians (now American Registry of Radiologic Technologists), and a longtime member and former chairman of the Commission of Technologist Affairs, American College of Radiology. From 1966 to 1972 he was a member of the AMA Residency Review Committee on Radiology. Dr. Soule is the author of scores of published articles.

GEORGE SZASZ, M.D., is associate professor of the Department of Health Care and Epidemiology and director of the Division of Interprofessional Education, Faculty of Medicine, University of British Columbia, Vancouver. Born in Hungary and having emigrated to Canada at the age of 18, he completed his premedical studies at McGill University and his medical studies at the University of British Columbia. A Milbank Faculty Fellow since 1967, Dr. Szasz has travelled widely in North and South America. In 1973 he was visiting professor at the Faculty of Medicine, University of Dar es Salaam, Tanzania. Dr. Szasz is co-author of *Adolescents in Society* (1968) and author of several publications on interprofessional education and the expanded roles for nurses and other health professionals.